IVF
DIET

THE IVF

DIET

The plan to support IVF
treatment and help couples conceive

ZITA WEST

Vermilion
LONDON

1 3 5 7 9 10 8 6 4 2

Vermilion, an imprint of Ebury Publishing,
20 Vauxhall Bridge Road,
London SW1V 2SA

Vermilion is part of the Penguin Random House group of companies whose addresses
can be found at global.penguinrandomhouse.com

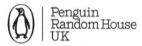

Penguin
Random House
UK

First published in the United Kingdom by Vermilion in 2016

www.penguin.co.uk

A CIP catalogue record for this book is available from the British Library

ISBN 9781785040399

Printed and bound in Great Britain by Clays Ltd, St Ives PLC

Penguin Random House is committed to a sustainable future for our business, our readers
and our planet. This book is made from Forest Stewardship Council® certified paper.

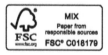

MIX
Paper from
responsible sources
FSC
www.fsc.org FSC® C018179

The information in this book has been compiled by way of general guidance in relation to the specific subjects addressed, but it is not a substitute and not to be relied on for medical, healthcare, pharmaceutical or other professional advice on specific circumstances and in specific locations. Please consult your GP before changing, stopping or starting any medical treatment. So far as the author is aware the information given is correct and up to date as at December 2016. Practice, laws and regulations all change, and the reader should obtain up-to-date professional advice on any such issue. The author and the publishers disclaim, as far as the law allows, any liability arising directly or indirectly from the use, misuse, of the information contained in this book.

CONTENTS

KEY TO SYMBOLS		
Egg friendly		Gluten-free
Acid–alkaline balanced		Diary-free
Sperm friendly		Blood sugar balance
Digestive boost		Detox
Immune modulation		

Acknowledgements

I'd like to give special thanks to our medical director Dr George Ndukwe – miracle baby-maker – Dr Simone Rofena, clinic manager, my great friend Anita O'Neill, and fertility nurse manager Terri Morgan Collins as well as the team of doctors, nurses, therapists and admin staff around me.

In writing this book, I want to thank Christine Bailey, the award-winning nutritionist and chef who has created the most amazing recipes, and Clare Casson, the amazing nutritionist at my clinic. Also my editors at Penguin Random House, Susanna Abbott and Morwenna Loughman and Julia Kellaway. And, of course, all my clients, from whom I learn every day.

Foreword

I have seen a lot of advances in the field of IVF since I first started doing it almost 30 years ago. The art and science have improved immensely, but I have come to realise that IVF is not just a matter of eggs, sperm and embryos. It takes two factors for a successful pregnancy – healthy embryos and a healthy implantation – and adequate preparation of a couple ahead of treatment is vital in order to optimise the outcome.

Our integrated approach to IVF at the Zita West Fertility Clinic involves looking at every aspect of a couple's lives, including preparation of the mind, body and spirit, stress levels and micronutrition, and diet is a huge element of that. It takes about three months for sperm to develop properly and slightly longer for eggs. Ensuring that they develop under optimum conditions improves the quality of the eggs, the sperm and, subsequently, the embryos. Healthy eggs and sperm equate to healthy embryos.

One of the greatest obstacles to successful implantation of the embryos and maybe the reason why IVF fails in some women is an inflammatory environment, which can be caused by autoimmune and other pro-inflammatory conditions of the immune system. If there is inflammation in the body, it could damage embryos and prevent successful implantation. At the Zita West Fertility Clinic we do specialist blood tests to see if this is the case or not. If inflammation is detected, we don't simply rely on medication to reduce this; the internal environment can also be optimised through appropriate nutrition and improvement in lifestyle. It is also extremely important to reduce the effect of stress, which can impact the immune system, and we use other, holistic treatments – such as acupuncture and hypnotherapy – to help with that.

Throughout my career, I have dreamed of being able to offer all these elements of successful fertility treatment under one roof, and this dream is now realised. I am proud to see it reflected in the wonderful outcomes and results we are getting at the Zita West Fertility Clinic.

Dr George Ndukwe, Medical Director,
The Zita West Fertility Clinic

Preface

In vitro fertilisation (IVF) and the medical technologies and advances that make it possible continue to astound me. I see babies born every day, yet still I find it incredible that humans have advanced to a point where we can create embryos outside the body and enable women who otherwise haven't been able to conceive to become mothers. I consider myself blessed to work at the forefront of this field.

Yet, at the same time, IVF, as we all know only too well, isn't a foolproof route to motherhood. It doesn't always succeed. That's why I caution all couples against relying on the science alone. If you are embarking on IVF, you must create for yourself the very best chances of success, and that involves taking a whole body view to the treatment you are about to have.

Lifestyle, stress levels and the ways in which we look after ourselves and each other are all part of my integrated approach. I am a great believer in Chinese medicine – an ancient but practical approach to wellness that enables us to see that all our body systems are interlinked, that nothing about the human body and mind works independently of any other. In this book I'll provide you with an overview of the IVF process and show you how to use your lifestyle and, specifically, your diet to prepare your body, mind and emotions for the IVF journey.

Fundamentally, I believe that one of the most important influences on a couple's chances of IVF success is nutrition. Everything that happens in our body is influenced by how we fuel it – with food from which hormones are released into our bloodstream. Never has 'we are what we eat' seemed more apt than for those who are about to embark on IVF. Good nutrition can support you and create an optimum environment in your body for the embryos to thrive. Good nutrition is fundamental to the health of all our body's cells, including those that go on to make eggs and sperm.

But don't worry, I'm not about to put you on some horrible restrictive diet. I want to take a realistic approach, showing you how you can use nutrients that are good for you in delicious recipes that you will love. In this way, the path to nutritional wellness for IVF doesn't feel like a chore or as if you're 'giving up' any of your favourite foods. Instead, I want it to feel like a culinary adventure to embark upon with great excitement. When you come across an unfamiliar ingredient or something you've never tried before, I urge you to buy it, cook with it and taste it. I promise that you'll love what you find.

All the nutritional advice is borne out in 60 recipes – each specially created for this book – that are easy to cook and intended for you to enjoy together as a couple. Remember that going through IVF is something you will embark upon as a couple, so spend time cooking together, eating together and talking about your lives, yourselves, your concerns and your celebrations while you do so. Strengthening your bond is such an important part of making your journey a success. It would make me especially happy to think that the recipes in this book had gone some way to encouraging closeness and communication between you.

When I opened the Zita West Fertility Clinic for couples going through the IVF process in 1990, I could hardly imagine the amazing variety of women and men I would meet, the incredible stories of strength and bravery I would hear, and the wonderful news of successes, of new families starting their lives together. I owe a lot of my success to them and the amazing team that I have surrounded myself with – many of whom have been with me from the start. Our doctors, nurses, therapists and support staff all share my vision to give clients the best possible experience and to prepare them on every level for IVF.

It has always been such a privilege to be part of so many people's most personal and intimate journeys into parenthood, and beyond. It is a role that I never take for granted. So let me know how you get on; I want to hear all your experiences of using this book and its recipes. I hope its advice is more than useful – I hope it helps make your IVF journey as positive an experience as it can be.

To find out more about our IVF clinic please go to: www.zitawest.com

Zita West

Introduction

I know that women love a plan. At the clinic we do too and we help you prepare on all levels at least four to six weeks prior to starting IVF. The very first task is to complete a questionnaire (one for a man and one for a woman). This takes you through key areas of your lives and your IVF journey so far, and provides me with both a medical history and a lifestyle/well-being review. From this I can create uniquely personalised plans. In fact, this is exactly what I spend most of my days doing. Broadly, there are three categories of investigation that we ask about:

1) **Medical**
   What you already know about your fertility issues re the blood tests and investigations you have had, the other tests you may not have had and still need. Looking in depth at your medical history gives us a clearer insight of how to plan your treatment.

2) **Lifestyle**
   Your lifestyle includes many factors that are often not taken into account when the medical side of IVF is the focus. Looking at work–life balance, alcohol, cigarettes and relationships, pressures etc.

3) **Mind and emotions**
   Here we get you to look at all aspects of your life to assess your stress levels and emotional well-being.

Of course, none of those categories works in isolation from the others, but by looking carefully at everything together we can create an individualised plan for each person (and couple) we see. Based on your questionnaire, we devise consultations to suit you and help you develop self-help techniques, such as managing negativity and your mindset, and visualisation. Consultations in the clinic include hypnotherapy, counselling and acupuncture, which is very valuable, especially prior to a cycle and on the day of embryo transfer (see page 205). Our nutritionists will assess you and advise on using supplements if necessary and the nursing team will support you all the way, responding kindly and sympathetically to your concerns and hand-holding as much as necessary.

Our aim is to enable individuals and couples to take back control of their IVF journey and to prepare themselves fully, on every level, for IVF treatment. We help you to focus on where your weaknesses lie with the aim of building up your reserves before starting IVF treatment. Looking outside the box to make a plan and pulling all the strands together is what we do really well.

The following are the ways in which you can begin to help yourselves.

DEVELOP A HEALTHY MINDSET

When a couple comes to me for help, the first thing I'm interested in is what is going on in their minds. What are they thinking? What do they 'feel'? What are their attitudes to their situation? What hopes and fears do they have beyond the obvious anxiety about their fertility? What expectations do they have for their fertility journey?

You're reading this book because you are thinking about or are already on the path of IVF. Like so many couples I see, your IVF journey is probably the thing that most occupies your mind. What if I were to ask you what else is going on in your life? As soon as you start to think about it, you'll probably realise that between you, you have myriad other demands on your time (perhaps a job, dependent relatives, house improvements, concerns about money, or even the toll of infertility on your relationship, among innumerable other things). Your mind is abuzz with activity. I feel exhausted just thinking about it!

Everything we do, eat, think and feel has an impact on our physical well-being. This is because the body responds to the environment we create for it. The messengers that tell the body how to respond are hormones, which, of course, are also fundamental to the success of IVF. Finding space in all that mental buzzing for some relaxation, some focused time together and some focused time alone will help you to cope with the demands of IVF and, in turn, balance your hormones.

TAKE EXERCISE

Exercise is a crucial part of physical and emotional well-being – think about how well you feel after a brisk walk or after swimming a few lengths in a pool. It's an opportunity to switch off your mind from everyday tasks and to improve your circulation in order to feed all your body systems with vital nutrients. Exercise has mental, emotional and physical benefits – holism in action!

MAKE TIME FOR RELAXATION

I encourage individuals and couples to use relaxation therapies for as little as 20 minutes a day. Not only is this calming during times of stress, but making dedicated time for relaxation helps us to build up energy reserves and emotional resilience, and to minimise stress levels in order to cope with the demands of IVF treatment.

INVEST IN YOUR RELATIONSHIP

Keeping in mind that you are doing this together is crucial to making sure the stress of the IVF process takes as little toll on your relationship as possible. Investing in your relationship could mean doing something as simple as planning time to talk openly with your partner, dedicating time to show each other kindness, finding strategies that mean you are supporting each other in the right ways (for each of you – no one-size-fits-all approach) throughout the IVF process or taking time out to enjoy each other's company away from thoughts of treatment.

Consider the opportunity to see a couples' counsellor if you are offered one – having an impartial observer to help you communicate with each other effectively can be really helpful.

PRACTISE OPTIMUM NUTRITION

This book covers all the main self-help approaches to optimising your chances of IVF success, each one having an impact on the health of the reproductive system of both the man and the woman, but most important of all are your diet and nutrition. The impact of ageing teaches us that sperm and egg health are themselves significant when it comes to improving the chances of IVF success. Healthy eggs and healthy sperm are crucial to healthy embryos; a healthy uterus, endocrine system and immune system lead to the best chances of pregnancy success.

Every nutrient and micronutrient you eat has an impact on your health, causing balance or imbalance, wellness or illness, depending on the nutritional choices you make. Every nutrient has an impact – however small – on the quality of the eggs or sperm you produce. Remember, especially, that a man's sperm is in constant production – what he eats directly influences this manufacturing system. This is why a specific diet plan, beginning at the pre-IVF stage and following every stage during the process is so essential.

Consider also that every other lifestyle choice you make on your IVF journey can impact your nutritional choices. Reducing stress levels, both through lifestyle choices and complementary therapies, and staying positive will help you *believe in* the efficacy of your treatment. If you believe and you feel in control of your life, you're more likely to make good decisions when you go to the cupboard to choose something to eat. However, negativity does set in after failed IVF cycles and you may look more at unhealthy choices (quick fix sugar for energy and eating fatty foods for comfort). Whereas if you feel in a better mind state and more positive and in control you are likely to make better choices all around and feel stronger emotionally.

Improving nutrition is a process – it's not something that happens overnight. I create a nutrition plan for my couples that means they build up levels of nutrients and micronutrients in their systems over the months before IVF treatment and during their treatment programme. The idea is that they are then able to optimise the health of their eggs and sperm over time. This book will enable you to put your own diet plan into action.

HOW TO USE THIS BOOK

The book is divided into five distinct parts, each one intended either to improve your knowledge about the road you're about to travel or to give you practical ways in which to improve your chances of success, including delicious recipes that are easy to make and full of all the vital nutrients you both need.

Part One (Understanding the IVF Journey) looks at the IVF process itself, beginning with the basics of fertility. You may know some of this already or you may need some clarification about information you've been given up to this point about how our reproductive systems work. I urge you to read it even if you already have a good understanding of what it takes to make a baby – lots of the terms (including hormone names) will come up throughout the book, so it's good to see why each of them is important in the context of a normal menstrual cycle and the man's cycle of sperm production.

Part Two (IVF and Your Lifestyle) takes a look at how your lifestyle choices and your state of mind can affect your fertility. I want to illustrate how helping to improve your chances of IVF success relies not just on your IVF drug protocol, the work of your clinicians or your diet (in combination or individually), but also on your mood and emotions. I believe stress (or lack of it) has such an important role to play in improving a couple's chances of having a baby and this part of the book looks at the ways in which you can help yourselves in your everyday lives. I see couples every day for whom small, daily changes in their attitudes, relationships or habitual patterns of thought could make a significant difference to their stress levels. This is my chance to share some of that knowledge with you.

Part Three (Preparing for IVF) is an introduction to all the nutrients you should boost in your diet along with recipes – as well as those it would be better to cut out or moderate – for improved reproductive health. We'll look at the role of supplements and the ways in which those on vegetarian, vegan and other special diets can receive all the nutrients they need. This section also outlines the diet you should introduce to help enhance your egg and sperm quality and improve digestion before your IVF journey begins. So much infertility is to do with specific conditions – PCOS, endometriosis and thyroid problems among them – and we'll discuss the nutritional needs of those with such conditions in this section. We'll also look at the diets of those suffering from intolerances and allergies, such as an allergy to gluten. Remember that your immune system can play a role in your ability to have a baby and allergies maybe a sign of overactivity in your immunity.

Part Four (The Countdown Nutrition Plan) looks at the changes you can make to your diet to make sure that, when the time comes for treatment to begin, you have established the best possible circumstances and environment for IVF success. You'll find detailed information and advice, as well as lots of delicious recipes, and a two week cleanse plan to help improve your hormone, blood sugar and acid–alkaline balance, as well as reducing inflammation.

Part Five (Diet and Your IVF Cycle) is where I will walk you step by step through the IVF process and show you how to adapt your diet and improve your nutrition to maximise your chances of success throughout every phase of the IVF process. For every stage, from stimulation to transfer, recipes and advice show you how you can use your diet for fertility well-being. At the end of the book, we'll round up with what to eat while you wait to take a pregnancy test. There's no magic formula here, but meal plans in particular can help provide a structure and some order to this agonising part of the process. At the end of this section, you'll find a brief guide to early pregnancy and what to do if IVF fails, including advice on all aspects of IVF; whether your attempt has been successful or unsuccessful, there is so much you can do to help yourself.

Part 1

Understanding the IVF Journey

My aim is to always give individuals and couples who come to see me the assurance that they have control over their IVF journey – so many arrive feeling that the whole process is happening *to* them rather than *with* them and according to their own choices. This section is about empowering you and giving you all the information you need – about your fertility in general, about the tests and investigations you'll undergo, about all the wonderful ways in which medical science can help you on your IVF journey, and about the IVF process itself – in order that you start out from a position of knowledge and understanding. This, I believe, will help you to ask relevant questions, make informed decisions and keep a sense of control over your IVF journey, every step of the way.

CHAPTER ONE

Fertility: The Basics

Most forms of IVF, to a greater or lesser degree depending upon the precise treatment you receive (see page 23), aim to artificially stimulate a woman's natural fertility cycle in order to increase her chances of becoming pregnant. In order to understand how IVF works, therefore, it's important to have a basic understanding of what that natural cycle is – including the ebb and flow of hormones that prepare a woman's body for pregnancy. Later you'll see that what you eat can have a significant impact on your hormone balance (see page 190).

A WOMAN'S NATURAL CYCLE

Hormones are chemical messengers that trigger certain responses in the body and tell it how to behave. The principal hormones that govern the menstrual cycle are:
* Follicle-Stimulating Hormone (FSH)
* Oestrogen
* Luteinising Hormone (LH)
* Progesterone

FSH and LH are known as gonadotropins and are produced by the pituitary gland in the brain in response to another hormone trigger – gonadotropin-releasing hormone (GnRH).

The ovaries store thousands of immature eggs, known as oocytes, within ovarian follicles. Every month, ideally according to roughly the same cycle, the pituitary gland sends out a pulse of FSH to trigger the eggs within several ovarian follicles to start maturing. At the same time, the ovaries themselves send out pulses of oestrogen into the bloodstream. These hormones work together so that only one egg becomes fully mature (in a dominant follicle) in each cycle. (If more than one egg matures, there's the potential for multiple birth – twins, triplets and so on.) Any other follicles that began maturing but didn't become dominant simply die.

The aim of IVF

Ovarian response changes from natural cycle to natural cycle, so you will have some months in which you're more likely to get pregnant than others. The aim of an IVF cycle is to ensure the ovaries produce as many mature eggs as possible, overriding nature to maximise your chances of pregnancy in every IVF cycle. IVF drugs mimic a natural cycle but provide hormone stimulus in larger doses than nature intends. The result is that, instead of getting one dominant follicle with one mature egg, all of that month's follicles mature, giving you several mature eggs from all of the stimulated follicles. Many women worry that this means they are using up eggs that they would have had available for other cycles. However, remember that in a natural cycle several follicles begin to mature, but (generally) only one becomes dominant with the others ceasing to grow. If anything, IVF makes use of those 'extra' follicles – they mature fully in an IVF cycle where in a natural cycle they would stop maturing and die.

Once levels of oestrogen reach a certain point, the pituitary gland releases LH to trigger ovulation: the dominant ovarian follicle releases its egg into the fallopian tube. The egg crosses a tiny gap between the follicle and the tube opening, and then is swept down the tube itself. Oestrogen levels then fall.

The empty ovarian follicle is now called a corpus luteum and this produces the hormone progesterone (and some oestrogen), which triggers the lining of the womb to become thick and cushioned, ready to receive a fertilised egg. If no fertilised egg appears, progesterone levels fall and the woman has her period. The first day of the period is an indication that the whole cycle has begun again. An IVF drug protocol uses synthetic forms of all these hormones in order to mimic the natural cycle.

If the egg meets a sperm and fertilisation does occur, its cells subdivide as it travels along the fallopian tube and makes its way into the uterus. By the time it's there it is known as a blastocyst and has many cells. If the blastocyst embeds in the womb lining, levels of progesterone (and some oestrogen) remain high in order to sustain the pregnancy. Cells that will eventually become the placenta begin to produce human chorionic gonadotropin (hCG), a hormone that tells the corpus luteum to keep on with its progesterone production to maintain pregnancy.

THE SPERM-MAKING CYCLE

Of course, men don't have a menstrual cycle, but there is a cyclical nature to the production of sperm. In fact, it takes two to three months for each sperm to reach the point that it is ready for ejaculation, although the process of sperm production is continual.

First, pulses from the hypothalamus in the brain release hCG hormones, which themselves trigger the release of LH (which stimulates the creation of the male hormone testosterone) and FSH (which tells the testes to begin sperm production) from the pituitary gland into the man's body. This triggers the production of sperm cells – the basic material the man's body needs to make sperm. The cells grow and divide in the seminiferous tubules in the man's testes. Eventually, after several weeks, they are known as spermatids, young sperm that have neither heads nor tails as we think of them, and are unable to propel themselves forward at all.

Only once the heads and tails have developed do the sperm make their way out of the seminiferous tubules into the vas deferens, a microscopic tube that loops and turns in a space that takes up a few centimetres in each testicle. The tube itself, though, is actually about 7 metres long! Unsurprisingly, it takes a while for the sperm to make their way through this tube – up to 20 days or so – during which time they are carried along by a sugary fluid that provides not only motion but also nutrients and energy, nourishing the sperm so they grow and develop. By the time it reaches the end of its journey, a fully mature sperm is primed and ready for ejaculation.

DIET AND YOUR FERTILITY HORMONES

The story of the menstrual cycle indicates just how important the rise and fall of each hormone is in order to create a mature egg and then to sustain it. Hormones also affect sperm production so diet is equally important for men leading up to and during IVF. In order for your hormone system (known as the endocrine system) to work both efficiently and optimally, your body needs to be generally in a good state of balance – and that relies fundamentally on the nutrients you put into it. A simple example of how diet will affect your fertility hormone levels is to think about fat cells, which themselves produce oestrogen. If there is excess oestrogen in the system because you are overweight (you have too many fat cells), you can upset the hormone balance that enables pregnancy to occur. Alternatively, if you are extremely underweight or undernourished, your body goes into survival mode, diverting nutrients and energy to support your vital organs (your brain, liver and heart, for example) and sustain your own life, rather than optimising the functioning of your reproductive organs. Simply, excesses are destabilising – everything should be in balance.

CHAPTER TWO

Starting Your IVF Journey

Before you begin your IVF treatment, you will undergo a series of tests and investigations to check for any underlying issues, such as cysts, fibroids or polyps, that might hinder IVF success and to indicate how likely you are to respond to treatment. If these initial tests are fine, there will be further investigations before your treatment itself can begin. (If you have already had failed cycles of IVF, you may receive tests that investigate why it may not have worked.)

TESTS FOR BOTH OF YOU

There are certain tests that both you and your partner will need to have in order to try to establish a cause of infertility and therefore to indicate which IVF treatment is most likely to bring a successful result.

The Human Fertilisation and Embryology Authority (HFEA) requires certain blood tests prior to starting a cycle, which include testing for sexually transmitted diseases, including hepatitis B and C, and HIV. The woman's blood will also be tested for immunity to German measles (rubella): this is because contracting German measles during pregnancy is very dangerous for the baby, potentially leading to miscarriage or birth defects. If you are not already immune, you will need to have a rubella vaccination before you are allowed to begin your IVF treatment.

TESTS FOR WOMEN

Tests for women usually begin with blood tests to check hormone levels. However, it is worth noting that some of these tests may not be available on the NHS.

TESTING FOR OVARIAN RESERVE

One of the firsts tests carried out is an ovarian reserve test as this indicates how well you are likely to respond to stimulation in your IVF cycle. The majority of clinics now offer women the opportunity to test for their ovarian reserve (the numbers of undeveloped follicles in a woman's ovaries). The usual test is for levels of anti-mullerian hormone (AMH), though an FSH test is also sometimes used. Unlike many hormone tests for a woman in relation to her fertility, the AMH test can be done at any time during the menstrual cycle. Because AMH doesn't rise and fall significantly according to any particular cyclical trigger, its blood level is relatively constant. Each test comes back with a reference range and a number which gives you an idea for your age where your egg reserves lie on the scale. High levels of AMH indicate good ovarian reserve, while low levels indicate poor ovarian reserve.

It's worth noting, though, that very high levels of AMH may indicate that you have a condition called polycystic ovary syndrome (PCOS; see page 134). If this is the case for you, your IVF treatment needs very careful monitoring because you can over-respond to the drugs you'll be given and can develop something called ovarian hyperstimulation syndrome (OHSS; see page 27).

Antral follicle count

Often AMH testing is used alongside antral follicle count (AFC). Performed in a clinic using an ultrasound scanner, this test counts the number of immature ovarian follicles (antral follicles) in both ovaries that are developed enough to be detectable on the screen. We know that women who have a high AFC show a good response to IVF treatment, while those with a low AFC show a poor response. Those with a lesser response are at greater risk of having an IVF cycle cancelled than those who have an AFC of 4 or more. The combination of the results of the two tests (AMH and AFC) gives a fairly good indicator of ovarian reserve.

Putting the results in perspective

Ovarian reserve testing (and the fertility potential your age appears to give you) provides only part of the picture – it may give you a sense of the *quantity* of eggs you have, but it doesn't give you any sense of their *quality*. A woman who is young but with a low ovarian reserve of good-quality eggs still stands a good chance of getting pregnant naturally. If you are in your 40s and your reserves are low, however, you can still become pregnant but the chances are lower. If you have a 'low' result, try to think of it as an indicator of what other tests and what sort of IVF treatment you might need, rather than an indication of certain unlikelihood to get pregnant. Nothing is further from the truth:

most AMH and AFC testing now is done as a guide as to how a woman will respond to IVF drugs.

THYROID TESTING

As we've already seen, everything in your body is interconnected. Rarely does the story end at a particular gland or organ. Your pituitary gland, which is responsible for producing two of the most important fertility hormones – FSH, which triggers the ovarian follicles to develop and mature an egg; and LH, which triggers the release of the fully matured egg (see page 8) – also governs the function of your thyroid gland. This small, butterfly-shaped gland in your neck is responsible for producing the thyroid hormone thyroxine, which establishes the rate at which you metabolise your food and your energy levels. Thyroxine is also essential for the proper functioning of your ovaries.

If you've been unsuccessfully trying for a baby for six months, having a blood test for TSH (Thyroid Stimulating Hormone) levels in your system can reveal whether a thyroid issue may be contributing to your difficulty having a baby. There's more information on this on page 136.

Thyroid and sperm production

Interestingly, some studies show that good levels of thyroxine are essential for maintaining good sperm production too.

INVESTIGATING PRIOR TO AN IVF CYCLE

Before your IVF treatment can begin, you may have several investigations intended to look at your uterus and ovaries. The simplest of these is an ultrasound scan, but there are other investigations that might also be considered:

* HyCoSy

  This is the shortened name for a hysterosalpingo contrast sonography (quite a mouthful!). It's a procedure in which a dye is introduced to the fallopian tubes via a catheter inserted through the vagina and into the uterine cavity. The ultrasonographer uses a handheld transducer inserted into your vagina to monitor the path of the dye on a screen. If you have a blockage in your fallopian tubes, the ultrasonographer will be able to see that the course of the dye is hampered in some way. Sometimes blockages occur as a result of damaged tubes, for example, of which chlamydia is the most common cause.

* **Hysteroscopy**
  A hysteroscopy may be performed under either general or local
  anaesthetic (which depends on your individual circumstances).
  A clinician will insert a speculum into your vagina (the tool used
  to open the entrance to the vagina when performing a smear test),
  followed by a hysteroscope (a probe with a small camera and light
  on the end). The probe is fed through your cervix into your uterus
  so that your consultant can see how things look inside your uterine
  cavity, and identify any abnormalities.
* **Laparoscopy**
  This is a surgical procedure performed under general anaesthetic.
  A laparoscope – a small probe, comprising a camera and a light – is
  passed through a small incision in your naval in order for a surgeon
  to assess the health of your ovaries, womb and fallopian tubes. A
  laparoscopy may be used to diagnose blockages in your tubes, cysts
  on your ovaries and fibroids in your uterine cavity, or other uterine
  problems, such as patches of endometriosis if this is found to be a
  possible cause of your fertility problems. The procedure usually takes
  between half an hour and an hour altogether.

In most cases, you'll be given the results of the investigation during the
same clinic visit (when you've come round fully if you've had a general
anaesthetic, of course).

Genetic tests

Our genes provide the coding that makes us who we are and govern the health
of all our body systems and all our characteristics. A genetic abnormality in either
the man or the woman (that is, an anomaly in the coding) may be responsible for
a couple's inability to conceive or for the woman's inability to sustain a pregnancy.

Genetic tests show inherited diseases, but also increasingly they are being
used to screen embryos for abnormalities that may result in the failure of IVF.
A genetic test can help to identify if you are an unknowing carrier of certain
inherited and life-limiting diseases, such as cystic fibrosis. Not everyone will need
testing and you will be advised by your doctors based on your medical history as
to whether you need them.

TESTS FOR MEN

TESTING SPERM

Known as a semen analysis, this is the single most important test that a man will undergo in the process of trying to establish any causes of infertility. Although instinctively many couples imagine that the problem must be to do with the woman's body, in fact around half of all cases of explained infertility relate to issues with the man's reproductive organs.

A semen analysis looks at different parameters for sperm health. The most basic analysis includes a count (the number of sperm in a sample), the motility of the sperm (how well they move) and sperm morphology (looking at the head, the neck and tail of sperm). Together these are reasonable indicators of a man's fertility. However, they are not the only indicators and it's better to have more detailed testing if you can.

SPERM DNA FRAGMENTATION

Even if a semen analysis shows that you have produced a normal semen sample, we still don't know whether your sperm shows any genetic damage – which can affect the success of assisted conception. DNA fragmentation refers to the proportion of sperm in an ejaculate that has DNA damage, which is increasingly becoming an important diagnostic tool.

If a man is found to have a high level of damaged DNA in his sperm sample, a clinic is likely to advise that the couple try intracytoplasmic sperm injection (ICSI; see page 28) over IVF treatment. If the sperm is really poor, a couple might choose to consider IVF treatment using donor sperm as a last resort, particularly if they have already had several failed IVF cycles without another clear explanation as to why this might have happened. Antioxidants from diet and supplements are thought to help to neutralise free radicals and so reduce DNA damage to sperm (see page 82).

MEDICAL WAYS TO IMPROVED IVF SUCCESS

The art and science of IVF have improved hugely both in terms of the treatment options available and its success rates, and there are myriad factors that can contribute to treatment decisions and the likelihood of success. The start of your IVF journey is all about investigation to make the chances of success as high as possible for you. A combined understanding of how fertility treatment can be tailor-made to help you and of how you can help yourself through diet, lifestyle and complementary medicine is key to optimising your IVF journey.

THE IMPORTANCE OF AGE
Certainly age is the single most important factor when considering your chances of IVF success. Quite simply, if you're a woman the younger you are the more likely it is that your eggs are generally healthy and the more likely they are to be chromosomally normal. Once you reach your mid-40s, your chances of IVF success are dramatically reduced. However, having said this, many women get pregnant in their early 40s and go on to have healthy babies. If you're a man, age affects the quality of your sperm even though production is ongoing throughout your life.

Of course, there is nothing we can do to wind back the clock, but there is plenty we can do to minimise the impact of age on the health of a woman's eggs and of a man's sperm. Diet is, of course, a crucial factor and that's why following the dietary advice in this book is so, so important.

Medical approaches will also take into account your age and do their best to maximise your chances of success. A range of tests and investigations, including tests for ovarian reserve (how many eggs you have in store), tailored drug protocols and specific age considerations taken into account during embryo screening, all aim to improve your chances of fertilisation and implantation success.

Heredity in fertility

Do you know how old your mother was when she went through the menopause? There is a hereditary element to the decline in a woman's fertility. If possible, ask your mum at what age her periods stopped altogether, then subtract 10 years – this is likely to be the age at which your own fertility will start to significantly decline. This can have an important influence on your decision of when to start IVF treatment.

Age and a man's sperm

Although men are constantly told it takes only one sperm to make a baby, the health of that sperm – for which age is a crucial factor – has a significant impact on IVF success. The use of intracytoplasmic sperm injection (ICSI) has greatly minimised the risks associated with age and sperm health, because it singles out the healthiest sperm for use in treatment (see page 28). However, there are also other medical interventions, such as intracytoplasmic morphologically selected sperm injection (IMSI, see page 29) and being able to check sperm DNA (see page 16) that further improve chances of success.

A couple's age

The younger a couple is when they undertake IVF treatment, the greater the chances of the treatment being successful. The sperm is more likely to fertilise the egg and the embryo is more likely to successfully implant in the woman's uterus. Furthermore, there is a lower risk of chromosomal abnormality occurring in the fertilised embryo, improving the likelihood of successful implantation and reducing the likelihood of miscarriage. A man and a woman who are fewer than five years apart in age, regardless of their age, are also statistically more likely to have IVF success.

Endometrial scratch Some clinics use this technique prior to starting IVF. The theory is that scratching the womb will stimulate an inflammatory response which is thought to help implantation. A catheter is inserted through the vagina to make a superficial scratch on the womb lining. Not all clinics will offer this to all clients. It is painful and you will be given a painkiller prior to undergoing the procedure.

THE HOLISTIC APPROACH TO IMPROVED IVF SUCCESS

At the Zita West Fertility Clinic what really sets us apart is looking at the whole picture of your situation, including aspects of your life that might be conventionally considered 'outside the box'. This can only be done with individualised treatments. I ask every couple, 'What do you want from a consultation?' The answer is invariably, 'We want an approach in which every aspect of our physical health, diet, emotional health, relationship and stress is looked at to optimise our chances: not just the science part.'

Fertility isn't black and white, there are many shades of grey. It can be hard for couples to take this in and to prepare themselves mentally, physically, emotionally and nutritionally for IVF: and this is where our approach to IVF comes in. Looking at stress-reduction techniques, acupuncture, mind–body connections, nutrition and lifestyle improvements, alongside the best medical practice is what differentiates us. My own experience of couples who have been treated in our clinic tells me that clinical and holistic approaches work hand in hand.

Can looking at blocks in mind–body connections and emotional imbalances really succeed where nature has not? Can nutritional changes and complementary approaches such as acupuncture, stress relief, relationship counselling, changes in work–life balance and so on really improve egg quality? In my experience, increasing a couple's sense of control over their IVF journey in this way does contribute to rates of IVF success.

So, I've introduced the concept of IVF, the pathways that will bring you to treatment and the basic principles of my own, holistic approach. Now you're ready to begin exploring the nitty-gritty of IVF and how you can use self-help techniques and nutrition to give yourselves every opportunity for IVF success.

CHAPTER THREE

The IVF Process

Making the decision to begin the process of in vitro fertilisation (IVF) is one that no couple takes lightly. On the one hand it provides a way forward, an exciting opportunity to realise your hopes for parenthood, while on the other it is an unshakeable reminder that having a baby is going to be more complicated than you might have originally intended. Arriving at this point is never straightforward – in order for IVF to be the next step, couples have been through myriad appointments, tests, investigations and results.

Although the focus of this book is how you can use your diet to improve your chances of IVF success, I want to begin with an overview of the whole IVF process – how your treatment will begin, who you'll meet, the different types of IVF and what you're likely to go through – so that you can put your diet and other lifestyle factors into the context of your treatment as a whole. I believe in an integrated approach to health and fertility in which the medical side, lifestyle and mindset work alongside one another during your treatment. This means starting from a position of knowledge and understanding how everything we do, think and feel resonates in our physical and emotional well-being.

FIRST STEPS TO IVF

There are two routes into IVF treatment. The first is through the NHS and the second is privately:

1) **Free treatment**
   NHS fertility treatment is free, but there are often strict criteria that couples must fulfil before they are able to embark on a government-funded programme. You'll need to speak to your GP about which criteria are relevant in your area.
2) **Paying for treatment**
   Paying for IVF privately adds another dimension to a couple's IVF journey. Having your own baby is, of course, priceless, but IVF is costly. It's essential to have all the facts about your circumstances

and your likelihood of success in place before you commit. Taking into account the medical facts, talk to each other about how much you can afford financially.

If you are eligible for NHS funding, you should consider this before embarking on a private cycle. However, paying for IVF often gives you more choices about the treatment, tests and techniques that will be available to you. Once again, start from a position of knowledge – know what your unique fertility situation is and look at all the options available to you (payable and non-payable) so that you can make an informed decision about how you want to proceed.

Money is itself an emotive subject for many couples. Agreeing between you what you're prepared to spend – or what you can afford to spend – on IVF is essential, but you must also be practical. Every day I see how difficult such a decision can be: it's rarely as simple as saying, 'We've agreed to have only one go at this.' Often, for example, the first cycle gives your clinic insight into how you respond to treatment. What you – and your clinicians – learn from this cycle can have a positive impact on a second cycle and, if necessary, beyond. Failed cycles often reveal the most important pieces of information for future success. Before you put a timeframe or financial limit on your attempts, try to make sure you have a full understanding of the treatment that you're likely to have and what it might tell you about your fertility journey if it fails. Once you have that information, plan ahead financially to give yourselves the best chance of a successful outcome without putting yourselves in a precarious financial position.

> It's important to set out with realistic expectations, not just in terms of your chances of success, but also how long the IVF process is going to take. Take a diary with you to your clinic appointments and map out a timeline of treatment.

KEEP COMMUNICATING

Embarking upon IVF is overwhelming and stressful for couples in so many ways. The fact that you both want to have a baby enough to consider IVF is testament to your commitment to one other. Managing your expectations is different for every couple and you will manage differently for your first attempt than, say, for your fourth. Prior knowledge of the IVF process will give you a good understanding of what lies ahead and how you can prepare yourself on every level. Keep talking to each other, respecting each other's points of view and listening to each other's cares and concerns. Accept that you may not always agree or see things in the same way, but don't let disagreement become a barrier to your communication about this journey you're taking together.

CHOOSING YOUR CLINIC

If you decide to undergo IVF treatment privately, you won't need a GP's referral – you can refer yourself to a clinic of your own choosing. (If you are accepted on to a government-funded programme, your GP will refer you to the fertility clinic in your area.) Every clinic will operate slightly differently and some clinics specialise in different types of IVF treatment.

Visit the available clinics during open evenings and you'll instantly get a feel for the place when you're inside it. Bear in mind that a good clinic should be willing to give you success rates. Online fertility forums can be a useful place to find out what other people have to say about a clinic and their experiences.

> The Human Fertilisation and Embryology Authority (HFEA), which governs practice in fertility clinics throughout the UK, has lots of information available on its website, including success rates for IVF for all clinics in the UK (see page 244).

YOUR IVF TEAM

Over the course of your treatment, you'll meet many different nurses, doctors, ultrasonographers and administrative staff. Knowing who each person is, as well as his or her role, is an important aspect of feeling in control of your fertility journey. If nothing else, you'll know who to expect to see at each visit and what questions he or she will be able to answer.

Your clinical team will include:

* **Your consultant fertility doctor**
  This is the person who will oversee your treatment, informing you of your unique fertility situation and appropriate IVF approaches. He or she will decide which blood tests and investigations you'll need (see page 23), which fertility drugs you'll take and when (your drug protocol) and what needs to change if you've already had a previous cycle.

* **Fertility nurses**
  Nurses at fertility clinics look after you throughout your cycle and organise and explain your tests and scans. They will answer many of the questions you have as you go through your treatment and liaise

closely with your doctor to implement your fertility plan. They will also provide crucial support. Your fertility nurse will be your first port of call for any queries or concerns. He or she will carry out tests, but also explain to you what each test means and ensure you receive the right level of emotional support, as well as medical care, throughout your IVF journey.

* **Ultrasonographer**

An ultrasonographer is a specialist medical professional trained in the use of ultrasound. Some ultrasonographers may also be midwives or nurses. He or she will use an ultrasound scan transvaginally to look at your follicles and womb lining, or to make assessments as you are going through an IVF treatment cycle in order to gauge how you're responding to treatment during your IVF cycle.

* **Anaesthetist**

The anaesthetist is responsible for delivering your anaesthetic to sedate you during egg collection.

* **Embryologist**

After you've had your eggs collected and fertilised, your embryologist will contact you either directly or through your doctor to let you know how your embryos are developing and when they will be ready for transfer into your uterus.

Throughout your treatment, your clinicians will do everything they can to optimise your chances of success. All the information you give, as well as the tests you receive, builds up a unique landscape of your fertility. With this landscape in mind, you'll be given a combination of clinical approaches tailored specifically to your situation. Your treatment pathway will probably include:

* Hormonal blood tests and baseline scans
* Blood test to assess your egg reserves
* Anti-mullerian hormone (AMH) and antral follicle count (AFC) scans to decide which drug regime will be best suited for you and how you are likely to respond to treatment
* Downregulation of your cycle at day 21 (not everybody will do this)
* Stimulation with injections to produce eggs
* Fertilisation of eggs and sperm – via IVF or intracytoplasmic sperm injection (ICSI)
* Embryo transfer
* Additional tests, screening and medications depending on what you and your doctors have decided prior to treatment

Importantly, remember that your entire team is on your side, aiming for the same, positive outcome that you yourselves are hoping for. Don't imagine that any question you have is too trivial or naive to ask – always seek clarification if you need it. The process can seem overwhelming, but you are in control of it. Nothing can happen without your consent – take your time, ask questions, make notes, and come back and ask more questions if you need to. No one will mind and, with a good team around you, everyone will support your insistence on making informed decisions.

UNDERSTANDING THE PAPERWORK

The HFEA requires that every fertility clinic keeps a careful record of the patients that pass through its doors – there are legal processes that need to be upheld and certain legal requirements for blood tests and consents that need to be fulfilled before you are able to go through IVF treatment.

You'll have a number of consent forms to complete before your treatment begins and even as you go along. Some couples find this unexpected and even overwhelming – the level of detail you'll be asked for can come as a surprise if you aren't forewarned.

Many of the forms are basic requirements of the HFEA. Additionally, each clinic will also have its own consents depending upon the treatment you're intending to receive. You will be asked whether you agree to let the clinic disclose information about you to your GP, who provides your ongoing medical care once treatment is over, but you do not have to consent to this. You'll also be asked whether you want to freeze embryos as a result of IVF or ICSI (see page 205), and there will be specialist screening documentation relating specifically to men and to women. Try to steel yourself for the level of detail you'll be asked for and take it one form or questionnaire at a time.

DIFFERENT TYPES OF IVF

In order for you to be able to tailor your diet and lifestyle to optimise your chances of IVF success, we also need to look at the different types of IVF and the specific tests and procedures that each involves – we'll go into more detail about what your body needs at each stage in the chapters that follow.

Many women I see, especially if they have had a failed cycle, arrive at our clinic having searched the Internet and already decided what type of IVF treatment is best. Often they are drawn to 'natural IVF' or 'mild IVF'. These are just names and IVF has to be appropriate to your circumstances;

some types will not be appropriate for you, while others will maximise your chances of success. Try not to begin with any preconceived ideas – it's better to get a full picture of your circumstances first.

Doctors try to use the minimum of drugs to stimulate you, but sometimes more are needed. Such decisions are based on your egg reserves and how you are likely to respond, so very small doses are needed in some cases and higher doses in others.

There are four main types of IVF: conventional, mild and natural IVF, and intracytoplasmic sperm injection (ICSI). Although there are features common to them all, each also has its own distinct aspects.

CONVENTIONAL IVF

This is the whole kit and caboodle of IVF treatments, but also with the most involved protocols. The most significant thing about conventional IVF is that, in effect, your natural reproductive cycle is artificially halted so that doctors can stimulate your body to behave in a precise way, according to precise timings. The sequence of events is usually as follows, although every woman and every couple's situation is different – not all stages and procedures may apply to you.

Suppressing the natural cycle

Your IVF treatment protocol begins with a two-week period (usually beginning on day 21 of your natural cycle) during which you will need to take a daily dosage of medication (a GnRH agonist) that prevents the pituitary from producing FSH and LH (see page 8), which would normally stimulate the process of ovulation. This is called 'downregulation' and it is not used on every woman: it will depend on the protocol you have been put on. You can usually administer your medication yourself, either as a nasal spray or an injection.

Sometimes the pill is used in the month prior to an IVF cycle to give the ovaries a rest to prevent cysts and to help with recruitment of antral follicles.

Stimulating egg production

Next, you'll be given an artificial form of FSH, (or a mixture of FSH and LH depending on what your doctor uses) which you'll usually need to take every day, for about 12 days, in the form of an injection. This stimulates several of your ovarian follicles to begin maturing eggs – more follicles leap into action than would normally happen during your natural menstrual cycle, meaning that more eggs become available for collecting.

Throughout the stimulation phase, regular vaginal ultrasound scans map the growth of your ovarian follicles until they have reached between 16 and

20 mm in diameter. At this size, the eggs are probably ready for harvesting and you'll likely be given an injection of hCG to mature the eggs and release or trigger ovulation 36 hours prior to the eggs being collected.

Egg collection

Collecting the eggs is a surgical procedure that usually occurs in the theatre of the IVF clinic or hospital you are attending. It only takes around 20 minutes and you'll be given a mild sedative and some pain relief in order to help you to relax.

The procedure itself should cause only mild discomfort (the amount of discomfort depends upon how many eggs are being retrieved) and perhaps a little bleeding afterwards. An IVF doctor usually performs this, not an embryologist. Egg retrieval is done using a vaginal ultrasound probe which guides a needle to aspirate each follicle; the length of time it takes depends on how many follicles are present. Once aspirated the eggs are inspected under a microscope and then graded by the embryologist.

Fertilisation

Shortly before your eggs are collected, the man (if you're using your own sperm) will need to provide a semen sample. In most cases the semen is 'washed' to filter out the healthiest sperm for introducing to the eggs. Within the context of the Petri dish the process is allowed to be as natural as possible – with sperm finding the eggs and attempting to embed within them. Sixteen to twenty hours later, your embryologist will look at the Petri dish under a microscope to establish how many eggs have fertilised, and will grade those that are.

Transferring the embryos

The embryologist will assess how well your embryos are developing and when they are at a suitable stage for transfer; this can be done on day 2, 3, 4 or 5. Both your embryologist and your doctor will keep you up to date every step of the way. Usually the embryologist will choose one or two of the best embryos from those available: the preference is for a single embryo to be put back, but if you are older more than one might be put back.

Unlike for egg collection, you are unlikely to need to be sedated for transfer. The procedure, which places the embryos into a catheter that is inserted into your uterus via your vagina, may be slightly uncomfortable, but shouldn't be painful. The whole thing should feel rather like having a smear test. The embryos are released through the catheter into your uterus and are left there to embed within your womb lining.

Sixteen days after egg collection, you'll be asked to take a pregnancy test. During this time – an anxious two-week wait that is often the hardest time of all for so many women – you may be asked to take progesterone suppositories to increase your chances of successful implantation, as well as other medications which may include aspirin and heparin depending on your history to help your body accept the embryos. If this round of IVF is unsuccessful, you'll need to have a follow-up meeting with all your clinical team to decide on your next steps. How long you wait before trying again will depend upon many factors, including how well you're coping emotionally with your experience.

The risks of multiple birth

There are greater risks associated with multiple-birth pregnancies – both for the mother and for the babies. This is why even if there are several suitable embryos available for transfer into your uterus, your embryologist will transfer only one or two. This can feel frustrating – it seems that the more embryos you use, the greater your chances of IVF success. However, try to keep in mind your end goal – to have a healthy pregnancy and a healthy baby. Multiple-birth pregnancy carries a significantly increased risk of miscarriage, premature birth and low birth weight, as well as pre-eclampsia (dangerously high blood pressure) in the mother. Your IVF doctor will look at your medical history and make a recommendation for how many embryos to transfer based on balancing risk with success. The aim is to put one back but this is decided by your IVF doctor.

Remember that everyone's aim is to give you a healthy baby.

MILD IVF

In mild IVF, a lower dose of drugs is used over a shorter period of time – working with your natural cycle – than in other types of IVF and fewer eggs result.

Ovarian hyperstimulation syndrome (OHSS)

Taking any medication is not without its risks and the same goes for fertility drugs, too. Ovarian hyperstimulation syndrome (OHSS) occurs when the drugs intended to encourage several ovarian follicles to develop and mature eggs during a particular cycle send the ovaries into overdrive: it is in fact a much less common occurrence as a result of more accurate ovarian reserve tests and more specific protocols. Lower doses of drugs help to minimise the risk. OHSS is an excessive response to stimulation that can cause symptoms ranging from nausea and pain in the abdomen to vomiting and breathing difficulties (which require hospitalisation). Caught quickly OHSS is perfectly treatable and your clinic will be monitoring you for signs throughout your treatment programme.

If you have developed OHSS you may not be able to have embryo transfer during that cycle. Instead, any embryos from the eggs of that cycle will need to be frozen and saved for a frozen transfer on another cycle. This enables doctors to get your OHSS under control, restore you to health and transfer the embryos at a time when pregnancy is far more likely to occur.

NATURAL IVF

This treatment is so called because it doesn't involve taking any medications in order to stimulate the ovaries or in any other way prepare the woman's body for collecting eggs. Rather, clinicians will monitor the woman's natural menstrual cycle and collect the egg that has matured naturally that month.

The process still involves an egg collection procedure (see page 26) and success rates for natural IVF remain statistically low. Since natural IVF relies upon monitoring your natural cycle, it is by its very nature relatively imprecise. It is suitable for older women who are poor responders to the fertility drugs and have a low egg reserve. While it is called natural IVF, some drugs may be used.

INTRACYTOPLASMIC SPERM INJECTION (ICSI)

When a man has a low sperm count, high levels of abnormally formed sperm (poor sperm morphology) or high levels of slow-moving sperm (low sperm motility) many clinics will recommend trying ICSI. ICSI follows the same IVF procedure for the woman, in terms of stimulating and collecting eggs, as conventional IVF.

In ICSI, the differences occur for the man. Rather than simply providing a healthy sperm sample from which an embryologist retrieves the fittest sperm for introducing to the eggs in a Petri dish, the man's sperm undergoes a careful visual selection process and individual sperm are injected into individual eggs to fertilise them.

You'll be asked to provide a semen sample at around the time of your partner's egg collection (often while the procedure is taking place or shortly afterwards), and then an embryologist will select only the healthiest looking and fastest moving sperm for injecting into the eggs. If you have a very low sperm count, are unable to ejaculate or have had a vasectomy, the sperm may be able to be taken directly from within the testicles – there are several procedures that can facilitate this depending upon your specific problem and your clinic will talk you through which is the most appropriate for you.

It's important to know that even with controlled injection into the egg, the sperm may not always successfully fertilise it.

Intracytoplasmic morphologically selected sperm injection (IMSI)
IMSI is a process where the sperm is selected using much greater visual magnification so that subtle sperm defects not as visible in ICSI can be identified (see page 210).

Single women going it alone and co-parenting women

If you do not have a partner or are two women in a same-sex relationship, you will need donor sperm, which IVF clinics will help you to source. If you choose to use sperm from a known donor there are many issues to consider about the role of the donor in your life. You'll need to seek legal advice before you start the process and implications counselling will help you to consider all the issues that may arise. If you choose an anonymous donor this isn't necessarily an issue.

Part 2

IVF and Your Lifestyle

When we talk about lifestyle, we don't just mean the areas of life that are commonly associated with poor lifestyle – drinking alcohol, smoking, taking drugs, eating junk food and lack of exercise. Lifestyle is about your whole life, including your relationships, your stress levels, your work–life balance, your thoughts and emotions, as well as your physical well-being. Everything within your body and mind is linked: your lifestyle is all of you, your way of life.

In this section we look at the lifestyle choices you make – or the reflections of those choices in your well-being (in your sleep patterns and weight, for example) – in light of improving your IVF journey. Many of the lifestyle choices you make will significantly affect your nutritional well-being, helping (or hindering) your body to make the most of the goodness you put into it. You can also use nutrition to improve your life and lifestyle: for example, certain foods will affect your mood and emotions. Remember that this doesn't have to be a great upheaval in your lifestyle; small changes can pay dividends.

CHAPTER FOUR

Transform Your Lifestyle

I try to ensure that every couple I see understands that collectively and individually they have lifestyle 'habits'. The term 'habits' is important because it helps cement the fact that lifestyle patterns are hard to break. So often, in their pursuit of IVF success, a couple will decide that everything in their lives must change in the instant they realise they're to embark upon IVF. They set to work with wonderful intentions, aiming for a 'perfect' lifestyle within a week or maybe two. Soon, though, they find the new, unfamiliar patterns of behaviour hard work. They might 'fall off the wagon' in some respect or another and berate themselves (or each other) if they don't reach their new goals quickly. I like to take a longer-term approach.

Changing your lifestyle is about consistency and sustainability, not instant perfection. Habits are habits – and new habits need to form over the old ones slowly, methodically and firmly in order for them to be long-lasting. IVF treatment is itself a long-lasting process, so the changes you make to the way you live your lives have to be sustainable. Don't rush. Take your time to embed your changes so that they become natural – even habitual – themselves. Cold turkey isn't the way. Give yourselves at least three months to effect change.

As a couple work through the following eight lifestyle areas (we look at them all individually or in combination in more detail over the remainder of this section) and think about how each of you can take specific, positive steps towards improvement. Make your goals measurable and achievable. Try to be neither vague nor over-optimistic – identify specific actions you can take, little by little, step by step.

Here are the eight areas to look at:

1. YOUR RELATIONSHIPS
We'll go into the nature of relationships and the importance of making sure you have good communication and support for each other, and in your wider social circle, in the following pages. Use the tips on those pages to try to ensure you embark on your IVF journey with a strong foundation beneath you.

2. YOUR ENERGY BANK

Before your treatment programme begins, you need to store up energy so that you minimise the likelihood of running on empty. All the steps you take to improve relaxation in your life, as well as improving your work–life balance, your nutrition and your activity levels, will help to build up your energy bank.

3. YOUR WORK–LIFE BALANCE

Related to your levels of stress and relaxation, assessing your work–life balance is an essential part of managing your lifestyle. We live in a 24/7 world, with emails, messages and phone calls in the palm of our hands. The boundaries between home and work are increasingly blurred, but few jobs are so vital that they can't be put down for an evening or a weekend. Learn to 'close the door' to your office both physically and metaphorically. Switch off your email alerts on your phone when you finish working for the day. Even better, turn off your phone altogether. As soon as you start to make this a habit, you'll realise that there's nothing that can't wait until the next day.

4. YOUR LEVELS OF STRESS AND RELAXATION

If you're stressed, your body goes into survival mode, shutting down non-essential processes, such as reproduction, and concentrating on the body systems that keep you alive. Nutrient absorption is hampered, hormones become imbalanced and overall your body is in a state of high alert. You'll need to take positive, specific steps to reduce stress and improve relaxation in your life. We go into detail about this on page 42.

5. YOUR MINDSET

Are you an optimist (always believing things will work out for the best) or a pessimist (imagining the worst)? Does your optimism need a bit of a reality check to manage your expectations (a positive attitude is a good thing, but not if it is delusional)? How can you bring more hope into your life if you're a pessimist? Take a look at pages 49–52 for some advice on how to bring more positivity into your life.

6. YOUR EMOTIONAL HEALTH AND YOUR MOODS

Think about how well you manage your emotions and how moody you are. What makes you feel positive and buoyed up? What saps your mood and brings you down? If you are the woman, are your moods and emotions cyclical? Perhaps related to your menstrual cycle? (Following the diet plans in this book will help to regulate your hormone levels and should even out symptoms of PMS, including mood swings.) How can you schedule your life to enable you to do more of the things that make you feel positive and fewer of the things that bring you down? How can you ensure that, as a couple, you support each other in your quest for more stable moods and emotions? Pages 49–50 will also show you how you can use food to help even out and boost your moods.

7. YOUR NUTRITION

Not only will you need to make specific nutritional gains in your diet, which is the subject of the remaining parts of this book, you'll also need to ensure you avoid anything that could deplete your body of vital nutrients. Smoking, drinking alcohol, recreational drugs and over-exercising are all nutrient thieves. Avoid them entirely (including over-exercising, although of course exercise in moderation is good for you) throughout your treatment – and beyond if you can. Once the habit is broken, don't reinstate it! Furthermore, your nutrition is fundamental to maintaining a healthy weight – and a healthy weight is in turn fundamental to IVF success.

8. YOUR ACTIVITY LEVELS

Lethargy is the enemy of wellness. Although it's important to relax, it's also important to exercise at appropriate levels. We'll talk more about this on page 51.

> ### Everything in moderation
>
> I am very frequently asked about smoking, recreational drugs, alcohol and caffeine.

RECREATIONAL DRUGS – WHEN ABSTINENCE IS THE ONLY CERTAINTY

Quite simply, nicotine and all other recreational drugs have absolutely no place in the lifestyle of any couple who wants to get pregnant – either naturally or through IVF. Studies show that recreational drugs such as cocaine and marijuana are damaging to eggs and sperm. Marijuana has also been shown to impact hormone balance in women, as well as cause early stage miscarriage. Cocaine affects sperm production in men and decreases libido. The story is similar across all the recreational drugs that have been investigated with regards to fertility.

SMOKING

Pregnancy rates are considerably lower in women who smoke more than 10 cigarettes a day. Nicotine is known to upset hormone balance and negatively impact the health of the ovaries and womb; not to mention damaging the development of a growing foetus.

ALCOHOL

Many couples drink far more than they realise. It is easy to stack up the units during the week, especially when you consider a bottle of wine is 10 units. No safe limit has been identified for alcohol with regards to fertility, but we do know that it can affect egg and sperm health: not only does it elevate the level of free radicals in the body, it also depletes the body of vital nutrients needed for reproduction. I feel, when you are doing IVF, you both need to give up alcohol in the weeks leading up to IVF and also during your IVF treatment. Some studies have shown that alcohol can reduce a couple's chances of successful IVF.

CAFFEINE

Caffeine is present in many fizzy drinks and painkillers, as well as tea and coffee. Studies into the effects of caffeine are limited but, again, when you are preparing for or going through IVF, it is best to cut it out completely.

Bear in mind that stimulants of any kind place stress on your body and stress depletes your body's nutrient supply, affecting all its systems, including fertility.

SOME WISE ADVICE

I want to stress that, in general, extremes don't work. Cutting out every indulgence in the pursuit of IVF success is not the way forward. There are some lifestyle factors that it's vital for you to cut out, such as nicotine and recreational drugs, but most of the time moderation is best.

One of the most important questions I ask my clients when they come to see me is, 'Do you feel that you're having fun in your lives?' So often the answer is 'no': a couple's lifestyle is not making them happy because it's too restrictive, and sometimes too accommodating (overindulgence makes us feel miserable, too). I firmly believe that lifestyle choices should make you happy, not sad. Leading a miserable existence, feeling guilty about the choices you make or frustrated that you feel you 'can't' do something interferes with all your body systems, breaks down communication between partners and increases stress levels. Don't look for perfection; aim to adopt good habits that are manageable, consistent and sustainable.

CHAPTER FIVE

Nurture Your Relationships

Like any major life event, IVF is as potentially stressful as it is potentially rewarding. Throughout your journey, your support network – from your partner to your family, friends and colleagues – will become an invaluable source of strength and stability.

FAMILY AND FRIENDS

I see many couples who are reluctant to talk to family and friends about their experience, as if articulating what they're going through somehow makes them seem like a failure because things haven't happened naturally or because they feel ashamed that they can't conceive. For some, though, letting in a few trusted friends is a relief, enabling you to be honest, direct and authentic when you're with them without the need for pretence when you're feeling low, stressed or worried. For others, IVF is an intensely private matter and many couples share their situation with no one other than each other.

In my experience, it's easier for couples to cope with the stress of IVF if a few, trusted people know about it:

* Your parents and/or siblings, who might start looking for signs that you're having a baby and ask questions about it. These are also the people who many couples find it easiest to call upon for support.
* Your best friends, who see you frequently, probably know your routines best and will sense when something is wrong and probably ask you about it.
* Your boss or a trusted work colleague who can ensure that you receive the right support from your company, including signing off the time you need for appointments and treatment without raising eyebrows. However, sharing personal information at work often presents the greatest challenge when it comes to talking about IVF treatment and lots of women struggle with this. Every manager, every workforce and every company is different. In an ideal world, you'll

find someone at work to confide in, but make your own decision about whether or not in the end it will work for you to have your colleagues know what you're going through.

It's also important to ensure that you steel yourself against comments that you may find upsetting both from those who don't know and inadvertently say the wrong things, and even from those who do. I've had clients whose friends have asked them which of them is 'responsible', as if it were someone's fault, how much it's going to cost or how long it's going to take.

Finally, even if you haven't told a soul, try not to withdraw from your social life or avoid seeing your friends. Especially those with babies or children of their own. This can be a common reaction, but in the long run it can have an adverse effect on your mental health. If you don't feel like being part of a big party, organise quieter social gatherings: a meal out with just two or three other friends or a long countryside walk with lunch at the end of it. It's important to keep plugging yourself in to life outside your treatment, to highlight all that's good in your life beyond your desire to have a baby.

YOUR PARTNER

Of all relationships, your relationship with your partner is the one you most need to nurture. Not a single one of the people I see in the clinic has the same viewpoint or outlook on their situation as another – including the person they're going through treatment with. No matter how close a couple or how committed each of them is to the treatment programme and to each other, putting in place strategies to ensure ongoing communication, openness and understanding is essential. Talk to each other and respect each other – always.

Remember that:

* Different personalities manage stress in different ways. Give each other 'permission' to express yourselves your own way, without fear of reproach. For example, men tend to be more optimistic about outcomes, whereas women see their own attitudes as more 'realistic'. Manage each other's expectations kindly.
* Coming to all appointments together is the ideal, but it may not always be possible and the reality is often very different. For the woman this can be very hard. Work together to identify those appointments where attendance for both of you is essential. Aim to go to everything together, but be happy if you only make it to those essential joint appointments together.

* Blame impedes worthwhile communication so do your best to avoid blaming each other for the situation you're in, and if you're the woman, try to stay focused on asking for your partner's support rather than becoming resentful at the thought that treatment is something that mostly occurs inside your own body. Equally, try not to blame yourself – remember that guilt is a form of stress, sapping the goodness from all the body's systems, including making it more difficult to take all the nutrient benefits from your food.

* Doing things together unrelated to your IVF journey is hugely important – keep the channels of communication open in your relationship by giving yourselves the opportunity for talking and even for focusing on something else in your relationship. Think about the things you enjoyed before starting a family became a priority and make time for each other.

* Your expectations and tensions will be changing according to the number of times you have been through an IVF cycle. Always be prepared to accept help from a counsellor. Sometimes talking on neutral ground to someone who can dig out the root causes of your frustrations and anxieties, and give you strategies to work through them together, is the best way forward.

Going it alone

Not every woman going through IVF has a partner. We are seeing an increasing number of single women, particularly those in their mid- to late-30s who haven't yet found the right partner but who want to have a baby. If you're a single woman, I strongly recommend you confide in a close friend or a family member to support you throughout the IVF process. Although it's your choice to have a baby using IVF techniques, the process is still a stressful one. This is especially true for women who have lived their life with the full expectation of meeting the right person to have a baby with, but for whom life had different ideas.

You'll need someone to listen to the facts with you, to hear them in their own way and be able to offer an alternative perspective or a checkpoint on the information you've been given. You'll need someone to help you pull together a plan of action, to help you to schedule your IVF journey into your life and support you at meetings and appointments. You'll also need someone to turn to if you do become pregnant (a family member or friend) – someone who can support you through your pregnancy and in the first days and weeks of having a new baby.

CHAPTER SIX

Build Your Energy Reserves and Reduce Stress

So many couples are told that IVF is stressful, exhausting and depleting. Preparing yourself for its demands and identifying strategies to manage the process can help on every level – mentally, physically and emotionally.

Imagine energy as a currency and you need energy reserves in your account before you begin your IVF treatment in order to sustain you through it. Many of the couples I see already have very low energy reserves and I see many women running on empty prior to starting IVF, juggling so many other things in their daily lives. It's important to stop for a moment and consider what's actually going on in your life. I don't necessarily mean your work (which I know you have to do), but what else? Are you building an extension on your house? Moving house? Organising a big event (a wedding, a big birthday party or a major holiday perhaps)? Are you looking after poorly or elderly relatives? Are you pursuing a promotion or trying to get noticed at work? Make a list of all the things that drain your energy and then start crossing off the things you can do without (for now at least).

Work–life balance

How much time do you spend at work? Be honest. I don't just mean in the office (or at your desk, if you work at home). What about the time you spend checking your emails on your smartphone, and even replying to them when you should be relaxing? What steps do you take to switch off from work at the end of the day? If you work at home, how do you mark the end of your working day? How do your contracted working hours compare to your real working hours? Start to prioritise your work–life balance. Stop checking your emails outside work – switch off your phone, tablet and home computer! Think of time-efficiencies that will help you get your work done within your working hours as often as possible.

I understand that life and work are all-consuming, but as couples increasingly fill every minute of their day, they are snacking unhealthily in order to keep going and never really taking the time to pause and enjoy a meal to its full. Think back over your week. How often did you sit down and savour your food at breakfast, lunch and dinner? How often did you skip a meal because you were too busy? How often did you just 'grab' something to eat while you were on the go? For most people, unhealthy eating habits (not just in terms of nutrition, but in terms of the ways in which we eat) stack up surprisingly quickly.

There are two things that happen as a result of this way of life. First, you don't give your body the reserves of energy it really needs from its food (instead you embark upon an energy roller coaster). Quick snacks, high in refined sugar and saturated fat, may feel that they get you through a slump, but ultimately they're energy depleting. Second, you don't give your body the time to restore its energy because you never pause. Make your IVF journey the impetus for change.

It's so important to make sure you replenish your energy while you're undergoing IVF treatment so that your levels are never too low. Remember, IVF is a stressful, whole-body event, drawing upon the reserves in all your body systems.

Women often ask me how they can build their energy reserves. Sleep is one obvious way, but also introducing stillness into your life (through simple acts such as walking in nature, practising meditation or mindfulness, or even just tuning out by listening to music), reducing stress levels generally and cutting out stimulants (including alcohol and nicotine) are all important energy savers. Your diet will play an important part in keeping your energy levels up (see pages 60–62). Many therapeutic practices (see pages 45–8) will also build your energy reserves.

SLEEP

The knock-on effect of longer working hours is reduced sleep and reduced sleep quality. So many people I see feel that they are 'owed' an evening, regardless of what time they stopped working. When they roll in from the office at 9pm, they eat late and are rarely in bed before midnight – they are then up by 7am the following day. Everyone's sleep needs are different, but in general you should aim for eight hours a night. Good-quality sleep is important and means you need good 'sleep hygiene'. This involves such things as making sure your bedroom is conducive to sleep (dark, cool, computer-free), your bed is comfortable, you have a consistent bedtime routine (reading for half an hour, say, or having a bath, then relaxing before getting into bed), and that you don't eat fewer than two to three hours before you try to sleep – your body needs this time to digest your food, enabling it to wind down rather than doing something active (digestion is an active process and disturbs sleep).

TAKE REGULAR BREAKS

How often do you take a break? From working, from chores, from your screen – in fact, from any kind of stimulating activity? We are all addicted to activity. I'm often horrified to hear that my clients take their phones or tablets to bed with them or spend their evenings 'relaxing' by browsing the Internet. I encourage my clients to schedule breaks. During the working day, every hour or so get up and do a lap of the office or, even better, a lap of the block (outside, in the fresh air). Take your lunch hour (or if you can't afford an hour, half an hour or even 20 minutes will do, but make sure you take it) away from your screen, your colleagues and your phone. Get out into the fresh air if you can and eat your lunch mindfully. Chew, don't gulp! At the end of the day, walk home if you can or at least part of the way home. Get off the bus or train one stop earlier and walk the rest of the way or, if you drive to work, do a lap of the block before you go into the house. Drink in the air. Make time in your day to pause and enjoy your surroundings or to focus on your thoughts (just 20 minutes a day is all it takes). Never, ever take your tablet, phone or laptop to bed. Say goodnight to your electronic devices long before you say goodnight to your partner!

Top Five Energy-savers

As you review your lifestyle, try to adopt these top five energy-savers that will not only help you to restore depleted energy, but create a much better overall work–life balance:
1) Get some fresh air every hour.
2) Finish eating your dinner by 8pm, then be in bed by 10.30pm.
3) Spend 20 minutes a day in reflection – you could meditate if this appeals to you or simply sit with your thoughts, watching them cross the screen of your mind.
4) Put your electronic devices – phone, tablet, laptop – away at least one hour before you intend to go to bed.
5) Eat mindfully (see page 106).

REDUCING AND MANAGING STRESS

The anxiety that is a natural side effect of IVF can often get couples locked into a negative stress response – when positive and good moments of life can seem all too fleeting and instead stress is an instinctual reaction to everything in their lives. I often ask my clients how they manage their stress and often I hear the answer that they exercise, in effect 'burning off' the excess adrenaline. Of course, there is great sense in that – it responds to the body's natural desire to 'flee' (see below) – but we need more than just exercise to reduce stress truly effectively. As well as exercise, we need to relax and to learn techniques that actually limit stress in our lives. Interestingly, very often when I ask women who've had successful IVF treatment what they felt made the most difference to the way in which they coped with the demands of their treatment, they answer that they improved their diet and they managed their stress levels more effectively from the outset. Women who have lower stress hormones in their system at the time of egg retrieval may have better overall IVF success rates.

Stress-busting foods

It may seem odd that what you eat can have a direct effect on your stress levels, but time and again science shows us that food can hugely influence mood. In fact, we know that the food we eat can trigger the release of certain stress hormones, including cortisol. There's more about this in the following chapter.

THE PHYSICAL EFFECTS OF STRESS

Stress is critical for survival. It focuses our attention, heightens our senses, raises our blood pressure and heart rate, and in general prepares us for the fight-or-flight response that can save our lives. At the same time, it shuts down systems not immediately important for short-term survival, such as digestion or reproduction. The problem with prolonged stress is that it can have devastating effects on the body, including on reproductive health. Chronic negative stress triggers a number of important changes throughout the body that act along multiple biochemical pathways, including the endocrine, nervous and immune systems. While we are all exposed to daily stress, when stress is severe, chronic or ongoing numerous biochemical changes overwhelm the body's ability to keep in balance. Studies have found that these harmful effects can persist long after a stressful situation has been normalised. It is therefore important you take steps now to manage your stress.

When we are faced with a stressful situation various chemicals – neurotransmitters and hormones such as adrenaline, noradrenaline and cortisol – are released into the bloodstream. They launch the initial fight-or-flight response in which blood glucose rises, blood vessels constrict, the heart races and blood is diverted away from the digestive system. Once the danger has passed, adrenaline and noradrenaline levels fall again, allowing the body to recover. The trouble is our stressful lives mean that cortisol levels in the blood remain unnaturally high for long periods of time. This can deplete our body of key nutrients and over time the levels of cortisol start to decline leading to signs of adrenal fatigue. When the adrenals become tired and worn out, our energy reserves fall. We feel tired and worn out, too, manifesting in symptoms such as depression, anxiety, low thyroid function, blood sugar imbalance, lowered immune function and sleep disruption.

Stress also activates inflammatory responses in the body and an increase in pro-inflammatory factors can have adverse effects throughout the body, potentially leading to muscle loss and low levels of key nutrients such as B vitamins, vitamin C and magnesium – all important for reproduction. In pregnant women, high levels of circulating cortisol have been shown to affect the developing foetus.

As you can see, stress is both bad for us in general and for reproductive health specifically. It's also worth noting that statistics suggest that stressed-out couples enjoy less intimacy and as a result have less sex – even when they're trying for a baby.

Cortisol and fat levels

Interestingly, studies show that prolonged high levels of cortisol can lead to increased levels of abdominal fat. People who are highly stressed for long periods of time tend to get more rounded tummies because the body thinks it's in danger and wants to preserve a source of energy (fat) rather than burning it off. High levels of abdominal fat can also increase inflammation in the body and are associated with insulin resistance. None of these conditions are conducive to pregnancy.

MANAGING STRESS FROM THE OUTSET

If you can begin the IVF process without allowing stress to take too deep a hold, you will have a head start on keeping things under control throughout your treatment. Use the following strategies to help you, but remember that implementing them in your life won't happen overnight. You'll need to keep reminding yourself that you're aiming for a long-term less stressed you and gradually they'll become second nature.

* Once you decide to begin IVF, you may feel overwhelmed by the amount of information you have to process. Be firm with yourself – tell yourself at the outset that you don't have to digest everything you're told in one go. Take things on board bit by bit, go back and ask for clarification if you need it and think of IVF as a journey. Once you accept that you won't necessarily be able to understand everything straightaway, you'll find it easier to be less overwhelmed and emotional about it all.

* Identify the major stresses in your life outside your IVF treatment – your work, perhaps, a difficult relationship with your siblings or something else – and think of specific strategies that will help you to minimise their impact on you as you travel along your IVF journey.

* Gather a support network. Who can you talk to about what you're going through besides your partner? Who makes you feel good and gives you a greater sense of well-being and positivity? Surround yourself with these people. Equally, who has a negative impact on your life, increasing your stress and sapping your feel-good hormones? Who would be best avoided for the time being?

* Learn not to overreact. Think of a trigger word to stop yourself in your tracks ('stop' is a good one) or count to 10 and take a long deep breath before responding to something angrily or emotionally. Give yourself space to process things and draw perspective before reacting.

* Stop the tyranny of the 'shoulds' and 'shouldn'ts'. There are no fixed rules; cut yourself some slack.

* Give yourself a break from endless list making. Lists feed into the 'shoulds' and 'shouldn'ts' and you'll feel shackled by them. Try to ease along with the process rather than fighting it or limiting it by making lists.

Supporting your stress management

There are plenty of therapeutic practices (see pages 45–8), including meditation, visualisation, deep breathing, hypnotherapy, yoga and acupuncture, that can form part of your stress management strategy. Try to dedicate 20 minutes a day to one of these in a conscious effort to bring stress management into your life.

Keep a journal

You'll need somewhere to keep a track of all your appointments, as well as a timeline of your treatment. However, it's also a good idea to have a journal – not necessarily with dates; a notebook will do, or even a private blog – where you can write down your thoughts, feelings and anxieties. Sometimes, expressing how you feel in written form is enough to relieve the burden of carrying those anxieties with you. You may want to share your journal with your partner or a close friend, or you may want to keep it private. You can use it to make notes of questions you want to ask at appointments as they occur to you (it's often hard to remember everything you want to say or ask when you're also being bombarded with information), and it can help you tune in to what's happening in your body, as well as in your mind.

COMPLEMENTARY THERAPIES

Many women I meet look to complementary therapy and practices as they embark upon or are going through their IVF journey. The term 'complementary' refers to the fact that these practices work alongside mainstream medicine in order to enhance IVF treatment. They give women a greater sense of well-being, help them to feel proactive in their treatment and encourage stress reduction. While there is both evidence for and against the efficacy (in scientific terms) of complementary therapies, there can really be no doubt that standard IVF treatment alone does not meet the essence of a woman's needs on every level. Consider drawing upon the wealth of professional knowledge and guidance that exists to support you, using complementary therapies, through the IVF process. Try to find techniques to practise at home: if nothing else, having a relaxation or stress-busting practice to focus on forces time out and away from either the busy-ness of life or thinking about IVF itself.

Our experience at the clinic shows that women and couples who draw upon the support of complementary therapies have a greater feeling of well-being throughout their treatment. We strongly recommend using them alongside mainstream medicine.

CHOOSING YOUR THERAPY

I see many women who haven't wanted to talk to their doctors about their interest in how complementary therapies might benefit their treatment because they know that there isn't enough scientific evidence to support their use. Sometimes we don't need evidence that something is going to work – we just need confidence that it will help us on some level, even if it is just to reduce levels of anxiety and restore hope.

The most important thing for any woman or couple is to identify a therapeutic practice with which they feel comfortable and a practitioner with whom they have a rapport. Next to making sure your practitioner is registered with a professional body for that therapy, rapport is everything, and there are so many excellent practitioners out there to support women through their journey at such a vulnerable time. Trust is also paramount – listen to your instincts. When you meet a practitioner to discuss the potential benefits of a particular practice, tune in to what he or she is saying to you and ask yourself whether or not you feel resonance between you.

I recommend that women in particular seek practitioners who:
* show empathy for their situation
* don't have firm or fixed views about when it is 'right' to start IVF treatment
* don't make unsubstantiated promises or claims about the efficacy of their complementary practice for the success of IVF
* understand the IVF process and know how to work with and alongside the protocols
* listen as well as talk, being led by the client's needs rather than steering the client according to the practitioner's own agenda

At our clinic, we work with three main types of complementary practice: acupuncture, hypnotherapy and counselling. These are by no means the only practices that can support couples through IVF, but they are those that we have found effective for all sorts of reasons over the years.

Acupuncture

I am fascinated by Traditional Chinese Medicine (TCM) and have worked as an acupuncturist for over 20 years. Acupuncture is a system of balancing qi energy – the subtle form of energy that TCM considers flows through channels, called meridians, in our bodies. According to TCM, illness (whether physical, mental or spiritual) results when energy blockages form along the meridians, impeding flow and upsetting the body's overall energy balance. In TCM terms, thoughts and emotions are linked to general health; and strong emotions such as worry, fear, anger and grief block the flow of qi energy. Acupuncture, the insertion of tiny needles into the skin along the meridian channels, releases these blockages to restore well-being.

If at all possible, we recommend beginning acupuncture treatment around two months before starting the IVF process. We also encourage our clients to have weekly acupuncture sessions during IVF treatment, with each session tailored to suit their IVF protocols. During this time the body can adjust, repair and rebalance.

Investigations into the efficacy of acupuncture have looked at its ability to improve blood flow to the pelvic area, reduce stress and improve IVF transfer. In my practice, I've known women who have become pregnant naturally during their pre-IVF acupuncture. We may not have firm medical evidence, but anecdotal evidence is sometimes all we need.

Hypnotherapy

I am a great believer in hypnotherapy and hypnosis as a means to relax, reduce stress and develop strength and stamina (mentally and emotionally) throughout the IVF process. Interestingly, one 2006 study in Israel showed that women who were hypnotised during embryo transfer showed a significantly greater likelihood of IVF success. It's thought that this is because stress at this point in the IVF journey causes the uterus to make tiny, almost imperceptible muscle contractions that may hamper implantation. If the woman has a means to relax fully during transfer and implantation, the embryo may improve the chances of successfully embedding in the uterine lining.

Find a hypnotherapist who can teach you self-hypnosis techniques to use throughout your IVF treatment (your clinic should be able to recommend someone or contact my clinic for recommendations). If the only result is that you have a means to enter deep relaxation while you're undergoing treatment, it will have been worth it.

Counselling

I meet many couples who are reluctant to take up the offer of counselling before their treatment begins and during it. Most say that it's because they don't want to seem to have issues that are affecting their clarity of thought or mental well-being in general. However, many couples, and especially women, experience high levels of anxiety before or during IVF. Having an opportunity to discuss their concerns in a neutral, confidential and non-judgemental environment can be very beneficial indeed.

Counselling is essentially a talking therapy – an opportunity to share thoughts and feelings. It's difficult to predetermine how it might be appropriate to you as there are so many options and scenarios, but I have seen it help couples with decision-making relating to their treatment and with working through the potential implications of their decisions (if you have opted for genetic screening, for example). If you're single and thinking about having a baby, or considering being an egg or sperm donor, you might also benefit from counselling.

There are so many reasons why the IVF process is stressful, so counselling can help to clarify your options and support you through your decisions. You can go together or alone; perhaps just once throughout the process, or maybe monthly or weekly. Explore all your options and consider every offer of professional support – even if in the end you decide it's not for you.

Strong emotions – from anger and grief to anxiety and fear – trigger a cascade of stress hormones in the body. Using stress management techniques for 20 minutes a day such as visualisation, hypnotherapy and yoga will help evoke a relaxation response which will help counteract stress. Another is to eat foods that promote rather than hinder good mood and to avoid foods that lower mood, and this is addressed in the next chapter.

CHAPTER SEVEN

Maintain a Positive Mindset

Your body is a wonderful cocktail of neurotransmitters and hormones, all of them telling you how to behave and how to feel. While your life circumstances have a profound influence on the levels of these messengers in your system, what you eat affects them, too.

For the purposes of this book, we're going to focus on two of the most important mood hormones of all: serotonin and cortisol. Serotonin is a so-called feel-good hormone, the neurotransmitter that tells you to feel happy, buoyant and at peace. Cortisol, as we've already learned, is a stress hormone, which depletes your energy reserves and lowers your mood. You can use your diet to help regulate these hormones in your system.

BOOSTING SEROTONIN

While some foods contain a little serotonin (for example, bananas), studies suggest it is difficult to raise your levels in the brain simply by eating more of these foods. This is partly because it is difficult for serotonin to cross the blood–brain barrier. However, one way we can naturally boost levels is to consume more foods rich in the amino acid tryptophan which is a building block for the production of serotonin. Interestingly, large amounts of serotonin are produced in the gut, a good reason to take steps to support digestive health.

Tryptophan-containing foods include:

* walnuts (and other nuts and seeds in smaller amounts)
* bananas
* plums
* kiwis
* tomatoes
* cheese
* eggs
* beans
* turkey
* seafood

In order to properly process tryptophan, though, and to turn it into serotonin, the body needs a helping hand in the form of carbohydrate. This helps the amino acids to cross the blood–brain barrier. Consuming a little slow releasing carbohydrate, for example oats, with a tryptophan-rich food, for example banana and nut butter, may be more effective. There's more on the best type of carbohydrates to consume generally on pages 66–7.

OTHER GOOD-MOOD NUTRIENTS

As well as tryptophan, try to increase the following nutrients in your diet in a bid to keep your mood positive:

* B-complex vitamins, especially vitamins B1 (thiamine), B6, B9 (folic acid) and B12, low levels of which have been linked to depression and low mood. The conversion of tryptophan to 5-HTP can be inhibited by a deficiency of vitamin B6 or insufficient magnesium, so make sure you are getting enough of these nutrients.
* Zinc is also needed for the production of feel-good neurotransmitters so include plenty of zinc-rich foods like pumpkin seeds, seafood, fish and lean meat in your diet.
* Omega-3 fatty acids have a role in the synthesis of serotonin and research suggests they can be helpful in boosting mood. They also help lower inflammation. Pro-inflammatory chemicals in the body cause greater production of enzymes that deplete tryptophan in the blood, which can result in serotonin deficiency in the brain and low mood.
* A vitamin D insufficiency may contribute to general depression so make sure your levels are optimal.
* Iron, which in low levels can lead to feelings of fatigue, poor cognitive function, apathy, irritability and sadness.
* Check your thyroid function – low thyroid function has been linked to depression and low mood.

It's important to say that we still need much more research on the delicate balance of macro- and micronutrients in the body and their effects on mood. So, while it's important to boost all those tryptophan-rich foods and to make sure you're eating plenty of carbohydrates, there's certainly no need to become carbohydrate-rich, protein-poor. Instead focus on eating a balanced diet (see pages 60–62) with an awareness of the foods that can help balance your mood. Note that during parts of the IVF cycle, increasing the ratio of protein to carbs will help improve the chances of success (see pages 152–61).

The role of exercise

We hear so much about exercising for weight loss and good physical health, but we rarely concentrate on the positive effects of exercise in relation to mood and emotions. You probably know from experience that when you have a burst of activity – it doesn't have to be formal exercise, such as running or going to the gym; it could be an hour cleaning the house, digging the flowerbeds or taking the dog for a walk – you feel better. This is probably especially true if your activity burst has happened outside (see below). This is because during physical activity the body releases endorphins, including serotonin (the feel-good hormone), which has the effect of elevating mood and reducing feelings of stress or depression. For this reason, among others – including maintaining a healthy weight (see page 53) – it's important to try to include exercise in your lifestyle in some form. Regardless of whether you should or should not exercise before IVF, some women need to as they feel very depressed when they don't.

Studies show that being in bright light increases the body's production of serotonin, which is why the impact of outdoor exercise is not only down to the physical release of endorphins in the body during the exercise itself, but also a result of being outdoors. A gentle stroll through the park, an outdoor t'ai chi class or simply sitting in the open air and watching the world go by will have positive effects on your mood and emotions. Furthermore, we need sunlight to manufacture vitamin D – which has a special significance in ovarian health and therefore for IVF (see page 69).

REDUCING CORTISOL

Certain foods in our diet have the effect of increasing blood levels of the stress hormone cortisol. Some of them are the foods that we already know are not good for us, such as junk foods that are high in saturated fats, alcohol, caffeine and highly processed 'white' carbohydrates. However, many vegetable and seed oils, when refined and processed to make them suitable for cooking, can promote inflammation and increase stress on the body, also raising levels of cortisol. Try to use light olive oil, coconut oil or small amounts of organic unsalted butter when cooking. Don't cook with extra virgin olive oil – light olive oil is less likely to smoke when you heat it. Extra virgin olive oil is best for drizzling or low-temperature cooking.

Fruit juice is another danger food. Although the fruit in itself is good for you, in juice form it is really little more than concentrated sugar. The all-round goodness of the whole fruit, which comes not just from the nutrients in the juice but also from the fibre in the flesh, is lost. Try to eat the whole fruit rather than drink fruit juice. Sugary foods (including refined 'white' carbohydrates) upset your blood sugar levels, giving you peaks and troughs of energy. During a trough, you'll feel depleted, low and hungry – all because the trough has triggered an increase in cortisol in your system. Chocolate is a well-known mood enhancer, but don't eat it as a snack. It's a treat, not a nutritious food, and I recommend only eating the bitter, non-sugary kind with at least 70 per cent cocoa solids. Low-fat (or no-fat) yoghurt can also be a problem because when fat is removed from naturally fatty foods, such as dairy, they become bland and unappetising. In order to boost their flavour, manufacturers tend to add artificial sweeteners and flavourings, so make sure you check the labels for ingredients.

Finally, always avoid foods that you might be intolerant to. Your immune response is directly related to your cortisol levels – if your immune system goes into overdrive, the body perceives stress and up goes the production of the stress hormones. Chances are you'll avoid these trigger foods anyway, but it's worth mentioning that you should be especially vigilant about your food intolerances if you're trying to manage your stress levels.

CHAPTER EIGHT

Lifestyle Factors That Affect IVF

Many lifestyle factors can hinder and have an impact on the success of IVF. Alcohol, cigarettes and stress are the obvious ones, but diet, nutrients and weight can also play a part.

YOUR WEIGHT

Being overweight or underweight can seriously affect a woman's chances of successful IVF treatment. However, I have found that it is rarely as simple as telling a woman that she needs to go away and lose or gain weight – often overeating or undereating are deeply rooted in psychological beliefs and behaviours. Women, or men for that matter, may overeat to fulfil a longing or a need, or undereat in order to punish themselves for a perceived inadequacy or because they feel sad.

WHAT IS OVERWEIGHT OR UNDERWEIGHT?

Conventionally the appropriateness of our weight is measured using a system called body mass index (BMI). Although BMI isn't the be-all and end-all of the story – where you carry your weight is important, too (apple shapes, carrying weight around the middle, are more likely to suffer hormone imbalance than women who are pear-shaped, for example) – it does give a good indicator of how your weight might affect your IVF success. BMI plots weight in relation to height – it doesn't account for your age or whether you are a man or a woman.

You can work out your BMI by dividing your weight in kilograms by your height in metres squared.

The following table will tell you whether or not you're a healthy weight for your height:

BMI	
Less than 18.5	underweight
18.5–24.9	healthy weight
25–29.9	overwieght
30 and greater	obese

If you have a BMI that falls within the healthy weight range, studies show that, in terms of your weight alone, you have optimum conditions for IVF success.

COMPLICATIONS FOR OVERWEIGHT WOMEN

There are many reasons why it can be more difficult for women who are overweight, or particularly obese, to get pregnant. Fat cells produce oestrogen which upsets the delicate hormone balance you need to fall pregnant. Oestrogen also interferes with the medications you'll receive during the IVF treatment programme, with overweight or obese women showing reduced rates of response to IVF drug protocols. If you're overweight and you have polycystic ovary syndrome (PCOS) – a common symptom of obesity – you'll need more careful monitoring and you'll be at greater risk of hyperstimulating your ovaries (producing too many eggs in a cycle; see page 134).

In overweight and obese women it's harder for doctors to retrieve eggs from the ovaries, largely because it's harder to get a good picture of a woman's internal organs. During the retrieval procedure, an overweight woman is at a greater risk of bleeding or abdominal pain and if she needs to have general anaesthesia, this itself carries greater risks for overweight and obese women (during any operation). Finally, overweight and obese women have a greater risk of high blood pressure, pre-eclampsia, gestational diabetes, implantation issues and miscarriage, among other risks typically associated with being overweight or obese and conceiving naturally.

Finally, being overweight or obese puts you at greater risk of Type 2 diabetes, which means your body can't control its insulin levels in order to manage sugar in your bloodstream. (Insulin is the hormone we release in order to metabolise glucose and turn it into energy.) Higher insulin levels have been shown to be damaging to a woman's egg supply. Also, fat cells produce inflammatory molecules and we now know that there is a correlation between excess fat cells, increased inflammation and a heightened immune response in the body, which may in turn have an effect on the success or failure rates of IVF treatment (see page 175).

COMPLICATIONS FOR UNDERWEIGHT WOMEN
There are fewer studies on the success rates of IVF in women with low BMI than in women whose BMI value is high. However, those that do exist show that IVF is less likely to succeed if you are underweight. When you're considerably underweight, your body goes into starvation mode. It believes that it must conserve your life and so channels all its nutrients and energy into supporting your vital organs, shutting down (through hormone control and release) reproduction as a non-essential body system because it imagines that it might be dangerous to procreate in famine conditions.

WHAT YOU CAN DO
In both cases the message is clear – do everything you can to bring your weight to healthy levels before you begin your treatment. Many clinics will refuse to treat women who are over- or underweight and will offer you nutritional and lifestyle advice to help you get your weight under control. It's important to see a qualified nutritionist if you're changing your diet with the aim of losing or gaining weight, and to do so slowly and sustainably.

Our relationship with food is complex, and to be told to put weight on if you're underweight or to take it off if you're overweight is often fraught with emotional issues. At the clinic we support so many women, especially with weight loss, not simply with dietary advice, but also with various therapeutic practices, such as hypnotherapy and counselling (see pages 47–8).

ENVIRONMENTAL FACTORS

We are all exposed to toxins every day in our environment. These have an impact not only on the environment itself, but also on our bodies, potentially causing disease and, importantly, affecting fertility.

Remember that sperm are constantly being produced in a man's testes, so his environment affects every batch as it's being made. For a woman, the eggs that are as yet lying immature in her ovaries are powerhouses of DNA switches that can be turned on or off, depending upon the environmental factors she's exposed to. Being considerate for and respectful of the environment in which you nurture your own body and your potential baby's is something that is as important long before pregnancy as it is during pregnancy itself.

There are three main environmental toxin groups that we need to consider when thinking about the quality of eggs and sperm and the likelihood of IVF success:

1) Plastics
2) Chemicals, such as cosmetics, cleaning products, pesticides and fertilisers
3) Heavy metals

PLASTICS: BPA DANGER

Plastic is an environmental nasty. Plastic containers contain chemical oestrogens that leach into the food or liquid contained inside the plastic itself. In scientific terms, these artificial oestrogens are a chemical called bisphenol A (BPA), which research shows can damage the chromosomal messages inside a woman's eggs. Not only that, but further research shows that BPA exposure may limit implantation success during IVF cycles (and natural cycles, too, for that matter).

Finally, any chemical that has the effect of mimicking oestrogen on the body will potentially affect sperm production. Oestrogen is a 'female' hormone (although men do have low levels in their own bodies) and an excess of it in the man's body may impede sperm quantity and quality.

What can you do?

Look for plastic products that are marked as BPA-free, particularly when you're choosing containers in which you intend to store food. Some sources recommend avoiding drinking bottled water from plastic bottles, advising water in glass bottles instead, but crushable plastic is usually already BPA-free (if you can concertina the bottle to get it into your recycling, it is unlikely to be made using BPA). Avoid putting hot food into hard plastic containers and check that tupperware is BPA-free. You should also ensure you always microwave your food in ceramic or glass (rather than plastic) dishes. When BPA-containing plastic is heated, the leaching effects are at their worst and even containers claiming to be BPA-free contain oestrogen-like chemicals that will find their way into your food or drink when heated.

DOMESTIC AND AGRICULTURAL CHEMICALS

Many cosmetics and deodorants contain chemicals that are harmful to our hormone system. Among them is a group of chemicals called phthalates, which research shows can affect egg quality and increase rates of miscarriage. You'll find these in some plastic containers (and terrifyingly in children's plastic toys), but also in cosmetics such as nail polish, as well as many of the products you might use to clean your home.

Agricultural chemicals come in the form of pesticides and fertilisers and are used in non-organic farming.

What can you do?

Go through all your cosmetic products (particularly nail polishes and fragranced lotions) and try and replace what you can with natural alternatives.

Eat organic fruit and vegetables as much as you can (a 100 per cent organic diet is ideal, but, if you have to choose, change those foods that most often crop up in your diet to organic). For any non-organic fresh produce, thoroughly wash and peel it before it is eaten or cooked in order to remove any chemical residue from the skin.

Finally, use natural cleaners in your home – products are readily available that are proud to say that they are kinder to the environment, which means they will also be kinder to you.

HEAVY METALS

In terms of heavy metals, studies show that lead will decrease sperm quality and increase the time it takes a couple to get pregnant, though the precise actions on the woman's body are still unclear. Lead exposure can also increase rates of miscarriage when pregnancy has been achieved.

What can you do?

Our environmental exposure to lead is mostly through our drinking water, where old piping was made from this metal. Many authorities now run schemes that allow you to replace old lead water piping through government financial assistance. However, if such a scheme is not available in your area, or if the cost of changing the piping is prohibitive, the most important thing is to drink filtered tap water or bottled water (from a glass or BPA-free bottle). Use filtered water for cooking, too.

Reduce your consumption of larger fish such as shark, marlin and tuna which may contain levels of certain heavy metals. Mercury in particular is linked to fertility issues which is why you need to be careful about the amount and type of fish that you eat in your diet. Instead choose smaller oily fish like salmon, mackerel and sardines. It is also important not to smoke and to avoid smoking environments as smoking increases levels of cadmium which can promote oxidative damage and inflammation in the body.

Part 3

Preparing for IVF

So far we have talked about the IVF journey in general and its effects on the body, mind and emotions. We've looked at ways in which you can adapt your lifestyle to optimise your chances of success and we've touched briefly on the role your diet has to play in that process. In this section we'll start to look at the specifics of how what you eat can affect egg and sperm quality, how to adapt your nutrient intake if you suffer from specific fertility-limiting conditions, such as endometriosis or PCOS, and how to make sure you get all the nutrients your body needs if you're vegetarian or vegan, suffer from food allergies or intolerances, or have other conditions that affect the foods you can eat.

CHAPTER NINE

The Importance of Nutrition

Optimum fertility calls for optimum nutrition. This doesn't mean some sort of punishing nutritional routine, but a sustainable, healthy diet that you can enjoy. I firmly believe that if you love what you're eating, you're far more likely to make healthy choices in your diet in general.

NOURISHING YOURSELF

Nutrition for IVF is about replenishing and restoring nutrient balance. It doesn't need to be complicated either – eating well is one of the most natural, instinctual impulses we have. Modern lives are often too busy and distracting for us to really listen to what our bodies are telling us they need. Short of time, we too often reach for convenience foods to stave off hunger. However, relieving hunger is different from nourishing yourself and your body – it's time to start really thinking about what goes into your body and using food to its best effects for the health of your eggs and sperm, and for your fertility overall.

In order to do this, you'll need to think of your body as a whole, all the systems working together for balance. This means your nutrition needs to optimise not just your reproductive system, including the health of your sperm and eggs, but also your digestive and immune systems; it needs to restore blood sugar balance so that you even out your energy levels and avoid energy peaks and troughs. You'll also need to make sure you have good levels of free radical fighting antioxidants in your blood, improving the overall health of your cells, and you'll need to restore your acid–alkaline balance in order to ensure optimum health in your gut.

The Mediterranean diet: a good balance

So much has been written about the Mediterranean diet and its health properties, and many studies into the best nutrients for egg and sperm health have looked at the Mediterranean diet. It seems that in terms of nourishing your body for fertility, we have a lot to learn from our European neighbours. No single food in any diet is a magic ingredient. Instead, we need to aim to eat a broad range of fresh fruit and vegetables, with good amounts of protein, moderate amounts of slow releasing carbohydrate and plenty of healthy fats (aim for omega-3 fats and monounsaturated fats, such as those found in olive oil and avocado; see page 65). I also recommend consuming whole milk and full-fat dairy (including yoghurt and so on, if tolerated). For cooking, consider using coconut oil which is rich in saturated fats and very stable when heated. You can also use a little olive oil for lower temperature cooking (for example, sweating onions).

Each day aim for:

- 5 portions of fresh vegetables
- 2 pieces of fresh fruit
- 1.2 g of protein per kg of body weigh (for a 60 kg woman this would be around 72 g of protein daily)
- 40 g of unrefined carbohydrates
- 2–3 tbsp of oil

TOP SIX NUTRITIONAL POINTERS FOR SUCCESS

Changing your nutritional habits, like changing any habit, will take time. The following are my top six pointers for successful nutritional overhaul:

1) Make sure you're both engaged in improving your diet: it's boring and time-consuming to have to cook separate meals. If you're both on board with healthier eating choices, you're more likely to sustain your new regime.
2) Manage your expectations: changing your diet doesn't mean you'll be pregnant within a week, a month or even three months. It means you're doing the very best things you can do to optimise your fertility for IVF success.
3) Understand the importance of digestion: take a look at pages 104–6 for tips on making sure you digest your food properly and for supporting your digestive process through diet itself.

4) Ideally, a well-structured, well-balanced diet (see page 152) will even out peaks and troughs in energy levels but, if you do have an energy dip, avoid reaching for unhealthy, high sugar snacks. Instead drink a glass of water or have a piece of fruit or raw vegetable and include protein in the snack to help stabilise blood sugar; for example, try eating a portion of fruit and nuts.

5) Improve your lifestyle: reduce your stress levels, spend time in moderate, gentle exercise, get outside as often as you can, manage your weight and improve your work–life balance (see pages 32–4). Remember that stress depletes the body of vital nutrients, so your lifestyle choices are key in optimising your nutrition.

6) Drink at least two litres of water every day. Your body can't function efficiently if it doesn't have water to lubricate its cells (which is why we feel lethargic and withdrawn if we're thirsty). Set a timer on your watch or smartphone to remind you to drink if you need to – keep sipping!

FOODS TO AVOID FOR EGG AND SPERM HEALTH

Of course, as well as boosting certain nutrients in your diet, for optimal nutrition there are certain foods, or foods from certain sources, that you need to avoid. These 'avoids' apply equally to both men and women. Cut the following from your diet:

* Trans fats (damaged fats often found in fried and processed foods), which damage cell membranes, increase inflammation and disrupt insulin function
* Alcohol (you should eliminate alcohol altogether during the pre-conception period – that means three months before you begin IVF treatment or begin trying for a baby; as well as while you're trying for a baby and in the duration of pregnancy)
* Fizzy drinks, which not only contain caffeine in many cases, but also high levels of refined sugar or sugar substitutes
* Refined carbohydrates, which means white bread, pasta and rice, as well as sugar in its refined forms
* Fish containing high levels of mercury, such as swordfish and marlin
* Foods containing high levels of omega-6 fatty acids – excess levels of these fats can promote inflammation (see page 65)
* Some overheated oils: overheating some oils damages them and 'feeds' free radical damage in the body

* Low-fat or no-fat foods. Small amounts of full-fat dairy or other 'fatty' foods contain valuable sources of fat soluble vitamins and are generally better for your reproductive health than the flavour enhancers used to make fat-free products more palatable

Foods for moderation

I am often asked about 'grey area' foods – those that are usually okay in moderation. Among the most common are: ham or ham products, which are fine as a treat, but contain high levels of salt; processed meat; smoked foods (again, these are fine as a treat, but be aware that the smoking process can increase free radical activity in your body); red meat (not more than twice a week); and chocolate, which for its antioxidant properties can be fine if it contains at least 70 per cent cocoa solids and you eat it in small amounts (not more than 25 g of bitter chocolate a day). Avoid milk chocolate or white chocolate altogether. Cake is fine as a very occasional treat, but it often contains high amounts of refined white sugar and flour – think special occasions only.

Finally, caffeine. There are all sorts of theories about 'safe' levels of caffeine, but my advice is to avoid caffeine altogether when undertaking IVF treatment or trying for a baby. In one study, women who were drinking up to five cups of coffee per day were up to half as likely to become pregnant as those who did not drink coffee at all.

EPIGENETICS

It is well known that your baby's unique genetic code is established at the first fertilisation of the egg in its DNA, which comes half from the mother and half from the father. Every organ and tissue grows from early pregnancy in a particular order and each requires the right nutrients at critical stages for optimum development. We now know from a branch of science called epigenetics that, while the pattern of development is determined by genes in the DNA code, there is a mechanism for switching individual genes on or off and adjusting the strength of their influence. It is apparent that the environment in which the foetus is growing can have significant effects on this mechanism and that markers can be laid down permanently that can positively or negatively affect the development of the baby into childhood and adulthood, and can even be passed to the following generation.

So making sure you have the right nutrition from even before you get pregnant is vital to ensuring that the nutrients are there ready for the baby as its needs develop during pregnancy. And equally, it is essential that any detrimental aspects of your lifestyle that might trigger an epigenetic response – such as smoking and drinking – are cut out.

MACRONUTRIENTS

The foundations of good nutrition come in the form of macronutrients: proteins, fats and carbohydrates. Each of these nutrient groups provides essential fuel or sustenance for the good functioning of all the body's systems. They form the bedrock, if you like, from which you can then tailor your nutritional well-being to especially support your IVF treatment.

PROTEIN

There are two main types of protein – complete and incomplete. Complete proteins are so-called because they are made up of all the nine essential amino acids the body needs to build cells and to manufacture hormones and neurotransmitters. All meat, poultry, dairy and eggs are complete proteins, along with some grains including quinoa, buckwheat, hemp and chia seeds, spirulina and soya beans (again, it is recommended to eat soya only once or twice a week maximum because of its hormonal properties).

Incomplete proteins exist in most grains and all vegetables. However, except for pulses and legumes, vegetables do not contain much protein. If you are vegetarian or vegan, focus on including a wide range of protein-rich foods in your diet over the course of a day, especially legumes, whole grains and nuts and seeds, in order to supply all the essential amino acids your body needs.

Proteins are the building blocks of your hormones and they are also so important for 'building' your eggs. This is especially relevant for IVF treatment when one is looking to increase the number of eggs available for fertilisation. Your ovaries need protein to mature ovarian follicles and release eggs during your monthly cycle. New studies on the success of IVF have indicated that women following a high-protein diet are more successful in conceiving. With this in mind, before starting IVF treatment we recommend an intake higher than the recommended daily allowance (RDA) of at least 1.2 g protein per kg of body weight. Some studies have recommended women actually consume more protein than this: up to 25 per cent of their daily calories (70–125 g protein daily) before starting IVF. To help meet your protein requirements you may find supplementing with a high-quality protein powder helpful (protein powders normally contain 20–30 g protein per serving). We have included protein powder in some of the recipes throughout this book for this reason. Having said this, it is important to focus on including good sources of protein (meat, fish, eggs, beans and pulses) in each meal, including breakfast.

FATS

So much bad press is given to fats, but fats are essential for the production of hormones and they provide essential fat soluble vitamins such as vitamins A, D, E and K. Beneficial fats include monounsaturated fats, found in avocados, olives and macadamia nuts, and omega-3 fatty acids, found in oily fish, walnuts, leafy greens, tofu, omega-3-rich eggs, flaxseed, chia and hemp seeds, and grass-fed meats. Saturated fats are crucial for the production of cholesterol, which is the precursor to hormones, so it's important to also include coconut oil and organic unsalted butter in your diet, in moderation. Avoid trans fats that increase the activity of marauding, cell-damaging free radicals promoting inflammation and insulin resistance (see page 62).

For IVF treatment (and fertility in general) the balance of omega-3 and omega-6 fats in our diet is crucial. Like some amino acids, these are 'essential', which means we can't make them in our bodies and need to obtain them from our diet. According to research, if the ratio of omega-6 to omega-3 is too high, there is a detrimental effect on ovarian function and the quality of a woman's eggs. Furthermore, lower levels of omega-3 can lead to problems with implantation, even if an egg is fertilised. Omega-6 fats are pro-inflammatory, whereas omega-3s lower inflammation.

Omega-6 fats aren't all bad though – we need them to produce prostaglandins, which are hormone-like substances that in turn balance the reproductive hormones in both men's and women's bodies, affecting sperm and egg quality. However, it is vital that we get the ratio of omega-6 to omega-3 right. Omega-6 tends to be high in modern day diets because we eat so many foods containing or cooked with vegetable oils. You can bring down your intake of omega-6 by avoiding margarine, sunflower oil, soyabean oil and corn oil. Instead, use light olive oil or coconut oil for cooking and focus on increasing your intake of omega-3 fats. Cold-pressed extra virgin olive oil is best for drizzling on to foods. You can also take a fish oil supplement to increase your intake of omega-3.

CARBOHYDRATES

A lot is written about the benefits of low-carbohydrate diets and some studies on IVF have indicated that a diet higher in protein and lower in carbohydrates is more beneficial for IVF success. This does not mean no carbs, but for good fertility health you need to keep your blood sugar levels in balance – there are strong links between blood sugar problems, insulin levels and infertility, particularly the onset of PCOS and ovulation problems in women (see page 134).

Rather than thinking about restricting your carbohydrate intake, eat good, healthy amounts of slow-release 'complex' carbohydrates – that is, carbs that release their sugars slowly into your blood, as a result keeping your blood sugar and insulin levels stable (see page 152). Slow-release complex carbohydrates have a low glycaemic index (GI), which means a GI value of lower than 40. They are unrefined carbohydrates: the wholegrain and 'brown' versions of the starchy foods we eat, such as rice, bread and pasta. Complex carbohydrates also exist in myriad different vegetables – leafy greens, Brussels sprouts and broccoli among them. Other low-GI foods include beans and lentils, and some fruits. The Internet has lots of sources for comprehensive lists of foods and their GI values.

Breakfast

Never, ever skip breakfast – it is essential for re-establishing balanced blood sugar levels for your day after the night's fast. The perfect breakfast combines both protein with a little carbohydrate and some healthy fat – think poached egg with vegetables and oat cakes – which will help you to feel full for longer and prevent unhealthy snacking before you get to lunchtime.

THE PERFECT BALANCE

Overall, your daily diet while you're preparing for and then going through IVF should contain:

* 25–30 per cent protein (or 1.2 g per kg of body weight)
* 30 per cent fat (about 65 g fat, made up mostly from healthy fats)
* 40–45 per cent complex, slow-releasing carbohydrates, such as whole grains or starchy vegetables like sweet potato, carrots and parsnip (about 200–225 g)

You should also include three or four portions of green leafy vegetables, and five to seven portions of other (multicoloured) vegetables every day. Finally, aim for two pieces of low-GI fruit (a portion of strawberries or a serving of melon) every day.

VITAMINS AND MINERALS

The knowledge we have about the nutrients for healthy ovulation and conception teaches us that a healthy diet that is rich in an abundance of vegetables and lean poultry, fish and meat is really all that we need to optimise fertility.

However, the reality is never that simple. Our busy lives mean that our lifestyle often depletes essential nutrients in our diet, exposes us to high levels of free radical damage and places a strain on our internal systems to rebalance the effects. Although lifestyle changes, as given in Part Two, will help to minimise the effects of stress and the environment on our nutrient intake, most of us will still need something more. Over the following pages we'll talk about the most important micronutrients (vitamins and minerals, in particular) that we need in small but essential amounts to give IVF the best chance of success. We'll talk about some of the main food sources that provide these nutrients, before we then go on to discuss the value of supplementation – which can give the body a helping hand when life and lifestyle stand in the way.

THE ROLE OF MICRONUTRIENTS IN FERTILITY

Increasingly we're understanding that micronutrients have an essential role to play in fertility, and by extension in IVF. Follicular fluid, which surrounds a woman's eggs, needs to be rich in certain micronutrients to feed and nourish the egg, particularly vitamin D (see page 69) and iodine (see page 72).

The following is a whistle-stop tour of micronutrients and their functions in the body (male and female) in relation to IVF. It's impossible to be comprehensive, but this will give you an idea of just how significant certain nutrients can be to your reproductive health and to improving your chances of becoming pregnant through IVF.

Vitamin A

This vitamin is essential for the growth and repair of all the body's cells. It also supports the immune system, is an antioxidant vitamin (fighting free radicals) and helps the body to rid itself of harmful toxins from the environment.

Food sources: oily fish (such as salmon), liver, cod liver oil, eggs and dairy. Your body can also convert beta-carotene (the compound that makes carrots orange) to vitamin A, so include colourful vegetables like carrots and other orange–red-coloured vegetables as well as leafy greens in your diet each day.

B-complex vitamins

It would be a book in itself to cover the enormous range of benefits of all the vitamins in the B-complex group. However, overall these vitamins help support all the body's processes, from cell growth to digestion. One of the most important B vitamins for reproduction, of course, is folic acid, which is essential for healthy cell formation and neurotransmission, which in turn helps to balance hormone levels. Another important fertility B vitamin is B12 (also called cobalamin), which not only helps the body turn carbohydrate into energy, but is essential for the healthy formation of DNA – the miraculous cells carrying our genetic information and essential for creating a healthy embryo. Finally, B6 deserves special mention as this vitamin has been shown to increase the luteal phase (see page 10) in some women, boosting fertility. Certain B vitamins like B12, folic acid and B6 are also important in lowering levels of homocysteine which, when it is high, can influence IVF success rate.

Food sources: B vitamins are present in a whole range of foods from seafood and shellfish to meat, poultry and game, and all the vegetables. Leafy greens, nuts and oranges are good sources of folic acid; pork, poultry, fish, whole grains, peanuts and soya beans are good sources of B6; and shellfish, salmon, cod, mackerel and eggs provide good amounts of B12.

Vitamin C

Commonly known as a great immunity booster, vitamin C also helps the body repair cells, metabolise important amino acids and absorb iron.

Food sources: red peppers, leafy greens, citrus fruits and other fruits, especially melon, tomato, blueberry, kiwi and blackcurrant.

Preserving nutrients in your food

The way we store, prepare and cook our food can have an impact on its nutritional benefits. Here are some top tips to ensure you are always getting the best nutritional value from the fruit and vegetables you eat:

- Make use of bags of frozen vegetables and fruit – quick and convenient, they retain good levels of vitamins and minerals.
- Don't overcook vegetables – quick steaming or blanching will help to preserve their vitamin content.
- As long as your kitchen is relatively cool, don't store fruit and vegetables in the fridge – many actually retain more nutritional value at room temperature.
- To improve the absorption of certain nutrients like lycopene (found in tomatoes) and curcumin found in turmeric, cook them with some fat, for example coconut oil, and add a little black pepper.
- Eat fruit and vegetables when fresh and ripe for flavour and nutrients.

Vitamin D

Our increasingly 'interior' lifestyles mean that vitamin D deficiency is on the rise. This is because the primary source of this vitamin is sunlight – the body synthesises it in response to the sun's rays on our skin. However, vitamin D is fast emerging as one of the most important vitamins of all for fertility. Studies suggest, for example, that it is present in the follicular fluid that nourishes the developing eggs in the ovaries and that women with low levels of vitamin D show an increased likelihood of implantation issues. Lower levels are also linked to PCOS, obesity and diabetes, and impaired immune function. Furthermore, scientists have found that the testes in men have vitamin D receptors, suggesting that it is an essential nutrient for sperm production, too. Sunscreen is important for blocking harmful rays, but it also blocks vitamin D absorption. If you can, try and get 20 minutes of sun a day with no protection.

Food sources: oily fish and eggs, as well as some dairy, fortified milk alternatives and mushrooms.

Vitamin E

We all need vitamin E (an important antioxidant) in order to help combat the effects of stress on the body, slow down the ageing process and maintain the health of our red blood cells. Like vitamin D, vitamin E is present in follicular fluid (see above) suggesting that it is another essential nutrient for healthy eggs. Studies show that it is also important for encouraging the thickening of the womb lining, which will help implantation. For men, vitamin E has been shown to improve sperm development and motility.

Food sources: leafy green vegetables, nuts, seeds, whole grains, avocados and wheatgerm.

Carotenoids

We've already mentioned beta-carotene as a precursor to vitamin A in the diet (see above), but this is just one of a family of carotenoids that give colourful fruit and vegetables their vibrancy. Essentially, carotenoids are 'just' the cause of pigmentation in these foods, but they are also present in the ovaries, apparently protecting them and developing eggs from free radical damage. Some research suggests that high levels of carotenoids in the ovaries leads directly to improved chances of IVF success.

Food sources: all brightly coloured (red, orange and yellow) fruit and vegetables.

Inositol

This nutrient compound was once thought of as a B-vitamin, but is now considered to be a nutrient in its own right and it acts like a carbohydrate. It might play an essential role in fertility and, in particular, in enhancing the IVF process because it stimulates the ovarian follicles, encouraging them to develop and mature. Furthermore, it provides the egg with a source of energy and it can help lower levels of the male hormone testosterone in the woman's body, improving hormone ratios for ovulation and fertilisation.

Food sources: unrefined carbohydrates, cantaloupe melon, oranges, most other fruits, nuts and seeds, and soya beans.

Calcium

It's well known that we need calcium to form healthy bones and teeth, but we also need it for good circulation. Some studies show that improving your calcium levels can help reduce instances of pre-eclampsia. Furthermore, calcium is present in semen, suggesting that it is vital in the support of sperm.

Food sources: dairy, eggs, leafy green vegetables, soya products, sardines and pilchards with their bones.

Zinc

Zinc is essential for the proper metabolism of carbohydrate into energy, as well as the breakdown of proteins into the amino acids that the body uses to structure its cells, and the enzymes that trigger myriad processes in the body, including the rapid division of cells in the fertilised egg. In men's health zinc is important for sperm development and motility, and is present in semen (see page 82).

Food sources: meat (especially turkey), shellfish, dairy, wheatgerm, nuts, whole grains, chickpeas and mushrooms.

Selenium

An antioxidant mineral, selenium provides support for the immune system. For men, selenium has been suggested to be important for good sperm development and motility (selenium helps the tail have a good, strong swiping motion). In one study, IVF couples in which the men were given selenium supplements, along with supplements of vitamin E, had a 10 per cent improved chance of becoming pregnant.[1]

Food sources: Brazil nuts, fish, meat and eggs.

Iron

Essential for the successful transportation of oxygen and nutrients in the blood, iron is also responsible for helping the body to metabolise protein and improve immune function. Some studies show that women who have optimum levels of iron in their diet or are taking iron supplements while they're trying to get pregnant have improved ovulation cycles. You can help your body absorb iron from your food by eating a piece of fruit for dessert, as the vitamin C in it helps the body with iron absorption. If you are concerned about iron levels, please get your level checked before supplementing as excess iron is not beneficial for the body and also causes constipation.

Food sources: red meat, green leafy vegetables, tinned fish (such as sardines and pilchards), whole grains, dried fruits, nuts and seeds, beans and pulses.

---

1 https://www.theguardian.com/science/2015/oct/20/new-dna-test-for-embryos-could-boost-ivf-success-rates

Magnesium

Women need magnesium in order to regulate their hormones, but it is rapidly depleted when we are stressed. Some studies suggest that magnesium might help maintain the smooth peristaltic motion that pushes the egg along the fallopian tube after ovulation, improving chances of conception. For men, the presence of magnesium in semen suggests that this micronutrient is essential in the support of sperm.

Food sources: dried figs, green leafy vegetables, whole grains, dairy foods, meat, fish and brown rice.

Iodine

Low levels of iodine have a proven detrimental impact on the functioning of the thyroid gland, which then affects all the metabolic processes in the body, but especially hormone levels. Iodine is also found in abundance in the ovaries and experts believe it is fundamental to the development of the egg within the ovarian follicle. It's also generally very important for a healthy pregnancy and baby.

Food sources: seafood and shellfish, and marine vegetables, such as seaweed.

The role of iodine in fertility

It's so important when you're going through IVF not only to ensure that you create the best eggs and sperm possible for fertilisation, but also that you create the most conducive environment for pregnancy to occur. Once any fertilised eggs are transferred to the womb, we want to optimise your chances of sustaining those embryos. Iodine deficiency has been linked with early stage miscarriage in women, so this is an important nutrient to focus on if you're embarking upon IVF treatment. Seaweed is a fabulous source of iodine, but so is saltwater fish (such as cod) and shellfish, and some dairy products. Iodine is also important for the development of a baby's thyroid gland.

But a word of caution: too much iodine can have a negative impact on your fertility especially if you have issues with your thyroid.

Carnitine

In some samples this micronutrient has been shown to improve sperm motility because it provides instant fuel, helping the sperm to swim faster and more efficiently. Furthermore, research suggests that men who had taken L-carnitine supplements for two months had a higher concentration of sperm in their semen than those who had not. It is also an essential source of energy for the egg.

Food sources: beef, pork, chicken, fish and milk.

SUPPLEMENTING YOUR IVF DIET

All of the nutrients described on the previous pages should come from our foods in appropriate quantities. However, when preparing the body for conception, and especially for a new round of IVF treatment, I believe it's vitally important to optimise chances of success by making sure neither the man nor the woman is depleted of any vitamin, mineral or other important fertility nutrient or compound. This is where supplements come in.

As a guideline, if you're going through IVF treatment and you are of optimum age for fertility (under the age of 35), the following should form the basic supplement requirements: a basic multivitamin and mineral that contains folic acid, vitamins B6 and B12, vitamin D, beta-carotene, iodine, zinc, selenium and omega-3 fatty acids, as well as other vitamins and minerals. If you're over the age of 35 and have been trying for a baby for a while, or are going through second or subsequent rounds of IVF, add in an antioxidant supplement, too (see our supplement range at www.zitawest.com). Specialist individual supplements, as recommended by a nutritionist at your clinic, who knows your situation, should be considered if you have certain conditions – for example, you may benefit from certain nutrients if you suffer from PCOS.

In addition, the supplements that follow provide a good base of further supplementation to optimise your chances of IVF success. Remember, though, that supplements are just that – they are an insurance policy, a means to supplement a healthy diet that is rich in all the vitamins and minerals, and all the macronutrients, outlined on the previous pages. The recipes throughout this book should help you to begin introducing these vitamins and minerals in delicious ways.

Begin your programme of supplementation at least three months before your IVF treatment begins, in order to repair and regenerate your body, and optimise your body's systems ready for IVF protocols.

CO-ENZYME Q10 (FOR MEN AND WOMEN)

Although it is not a vitamin, co-enzyme Q10 (co-Q10) acts like one and it is produced within every cell of the body. It both protects our cells (it is an antioxidant) and is a trigger for their function. It provides a source of fuel for the mitochondria cells that power the sperm and provide energy for the egg in its incredible and rapid subdivision after fertilisation. Not only that, some studies suggest that good levels of co-Q10 promote the development of eggs within the ovarian follicles, improving the chances of more eggs reaching full maturity, which is why it is so important for women undergoing IVF. In men, its antioxidant and energy-giving powers are generally good news for sperm health and production and so is included in some supplements.

MELATONIN (FOR WOMEN)

Naturally produced, this is the hormone that regulates our body clock, telling us when to shut down for sleep (you may have heard it referred to as the 'sleep hormone'). Interestingly, it also increases oestrogen sensitivity in the ovaries and uterine lining in women, improving ovulation and implantation rates. In IVF treatment, studies have shown that women taking melatonin supplements produce more good eggs that are successfully fertilised. Please note that melatonin is not available as a supplement in the UK, although it is available if needed on prescription.

DEHYDROEPIANDROSTERONE (FOR MEN AND WOMEN)

Dehydroepiandrosterone (DHEA) is a precursor hormone produced naturally in the adrenal glands and brain in both men and women, and in the testes in men. It has strong links with sexual function and reproduction because it is the precursor for testosterone (an androgen, or male hormone) and oestrogen.

DHEA supplements need to be taken with caution as they can convert to oestrogen or testosterone in the body and damage eggs. Supplementation of this hormone should be under careful guidance from your medical practitioner as in its artificial, supplement form it has side effects that include hair loss and acne. If you have a past history of fibroids you shouldn't take DHEA, so please seek specialist advice from your doctor before taking this supplement.

N-ACETYL CYSTEINE

An amino acid, N-acetyl cysteine (NAC) has been shown to improve egg quality in women with PCOS, improve insulin sensitivity and help to reduce inflammation in the body – all of which can have a positive effect on the rates of IVF success. Furthermore, some scientists believe NAC can even protect the health of the ovaries, reducing incidence of cell damage through things such as free radicals.

PHOSPHOLIPIDS

Phospholipids are a group of fats that will help protect and repair cell membranes and help with the modulation of the immune system. Look for a supplement powder that contains phosphatidic acid, phosphatidyl choline, phosphatidyl ethanolamine, phosphatidyl glycerol and phosphatidyl serine.

Every client, every couple and every situation is different, so it seems inappropriate to generalise about how much of each of these supplements you should take in order to improve your chances of IVF success. Talk to your clinic's nutritional consultant about appropriate levels of supplementation for your situation.

CHAPTER TEN

Egg and Sperm Health

NOURISHING YOUR EGGS

The single most frequently asked question among women undergoing IVF treatment is, 'What can I do to improve the quality of my eggs?' One answer is, 'Optimise your egg-friendly nutrition.'

Although it's true that you are born with all the eggs you will ever have, the quality of your eggs is not fixed. The environment you create for your developing eggs is crucial when it comes to making sure that they are genetically as healthy as they can be. Age is, of course, the biggest factor affecting egg quality but, if you are older, you need to feel that you are doing everything you can to make that environment the best it can be. Lifestyle, diet and nutrition can all play a part in this.

Healthy DNA (the molecules that contain our genetic information) means chromosomally normal eggs, which stand a greater chance of being receptive to fertilisation by a sperm. The cells of a healthy egg are also more likely to divide normally once it's fertilised and to create an embryo (or blastocyst in the very early stages) that will implant in the womb.

The quality of your eggs is paramount.

THE HUMAN EGG

There are four principal layers in a human egg:

1) **Corona radiate**
   The outermost layer, the corona radiate is made up of layers of cells taken from the ovarian follicle. These cells provide nourishment (in the form of proteins) for the other layers of the egg.
2) **Zona pellucida**
   A membrane that surrounds and protects the innermost part of the egg, the zona pellucida is the 'shell'. It is made up of fats known as lipids and phospholipids and it allows the passage of nutrients into and out of the egg. The zona pellucida gets harder with age, making it more difficult for sperm to penetrate and for a fertilised egg to implant. Finally, free radicals (marauding, unstable cells) can damage

the zona pellucida, which in turn can mean damage to mitochondrial function within the next cell layer (see below).

3) Cytoplasm

Lots of people refer to this gelatinous layer of the human egg as our 'yolk'. Made up mainly of water and salt, the cytoplasm is the main energy source of the egg cell. It contains special 'organelles' called mitochondria, which are amazing powerhouses of energy that take nutrients and oxygen from the cell wall and metabolise them so that the cell can use them to function. The human egg has one of the highest concentrations of mitochondria in its cytoplasm of any cell in the human body and good nutrition is essential to deliver its energy.

4) Nucleus

This innermost layer of the human egg stores all of its genetic information. Here, 23 chromosomes (half the number we need to make a genetically normal baby; the other half coming from the sperm) contain thousands of pieces of DNA information that will help determine everything from the baby's hair colour to his or her left- or right-handedness. Although all the information is there, DNA needs activation – switching on or off in myriad permutations and combinations. The environment – including how we feed our bodies – we create for these latent pieces of information can determine which genes are activated and which are not. The biggest factor affecting the DNA inside the nucleus of the egg is age, so eating to preserve the health of your eggs is paramount.

It takes approximately 150 days for an egg to mature within its ovarian follicle. This means there are four months during which you have an opportunity to nourish any single month's particular crop. Some of the eggs that begin to mature will not make it to full maturity, but one – and perhaps more – will. Health (and damage) can occur along the way, with the Meiosis 1 stage of maturation being the most important. This is the point just before ovulation when cells within the nucleus become the all-important 23 chromosomes that will provide half the baby's genetic information.

There is a single, important message here – your nutritional choices and your lifestyle choices may improve the quality of your eggs, but it will take time. If you start changing your diet today, the impact will likely be most significant on eggs that your body is maturing for release in four months' time. However, if the point just before ovulation is most important in terms of determining the chromosomal health of a single, mature egg, the impact of what you put into your body may be as immediate as next month's reproductive cycle. It's never too soon, nor too late. to begin making improvements to your diet.

IMPROVING THE QUALITY OF YOUR EGGS

So, what do your eggs need from your diet in order to be the best they can be?

1) **Energy**

   The main source of energy in your diet is sugar. However, as we already know sugar comes in different forms. The best type of sugar for cell metabolism comes from unrefined carbohydrates – brown and wholegrain starches that release energy slowly into the body. Furthermore, foods rich in co-enzyme Q10 (see page 80), a nutrient especially rich in oily fish, beef and poultry, helps with the metabolism of nutrients to turn them into energy. In addition, try to eat foods rich in inositol, a carbohydrate-like nutrient that helps with the transfer of energy and nutrients into and out of the body's cells.

Inositol

Inositol is part of the B vitamin family and has been found in the follicular fluid of higher quality eggs. Increasingly evidence suggests the use of inositol may help mature eggs during an IVF cycle and is needed in follicular fluid which surrounds the eggs taken prior to an IVF cycle. Inositol is found in high-fibre, unrefined foods, as well as leafy greens, bananas, cantaloupe melon, citrus fruits, nuts and seeds, lecithin granules and soya beans. (I recommend eating soya only once or twice a week maximum because of its hormonal properties.) Try including 1–2 tsp (approx. 4 g) of inositol daily in your diet. This is an available Zita West product.

---

2) **Fats**

   Because the zona pellucida is made up of fats, and because fats help to improve the metabolism of nutrients to energy, foods rich in omega-3 and -6 fatty acids (in the right balance; see page 65), as well as other polyunsaturated fats, are an important part of an egg-friendly diet.

3) **Protein**

   Found primarily in dairy, pulses, poultry, meat and fish, proteins are the building blocks of all the cells in the body.

4) **Micronutrients**

   As well as co-enzyme Q10 (see above) other micronutrients among the most important are: zinc, vitamin D, beta-carotene (which the body converts to vitamin A) and iodine.

5) Antioxidants

These are natural free radical beaters, helping to protect our cells from DNA damage. Antioxidants are found in brightly coloured fruit and vegetables. Vitamins A, C and E (the ACE vitamins) are particularly brilliant antioxidants, as are zinc, selenium and magnesium and, again, co-enzyme Q10. These are all good immunity-protectors, too, and a strong immune system is another important factor when protecting the health of your eggs (see page 175).

6) Hormone-balancing foods

It stands to reason that healthy eggs are the product of well-balanced hormones – the chemical triggers that tell the body what to do and how to develop. There are many lifestyle choices that will affect hormone levels, including reducing stress and stabilising energy levels, but diet is important too. If you wish to eat meat, choose grass-fed organic meat and organic dairy products. You can also include foods that help excretion and balance of hormones, such as flaxseed.

Finally, remember that balance in all things is key.

YOUR AGE

We already know that the single most important factor when it comes to fertility success is the quality of the eggs and sperm that make a baby. A woman's age, in particular, affects egg quality, with eggs in an older woman more likely to have chromosomal defects and therefore be less suitable for fertilisation.

However, I firmly believe there is so much a woman can do nutritionally to improve the quality of her eggs, even when she is beyond the age of 35 or even 40, and I am so heartened when I hear that older women have become pregnant against the odds.

Antioxidants, antioxidants, antioxidants

Cell-ageing – whether that's in the cells of the skin, the internal organs, a sperm or a developing egg within an ovarian follicle – is the result of the action of free radicals. Stable atoms and molecules in our body are made up of pairs of electrons. A free radical has a random, unpaired electron, making it unstable and dangerous to other cells. It zips around the body with the aim of stealing an electron (in a process called oxidation) from a healthy cell, thereby damaging that cell's function irreparably.

Free radical damage is an unavoidable and completely natural by-product of our metabolism. However, we can also accelerate it by eating unhealthily (having a diet high in saturated fat and junk foods, for example), drinking alcohol, taking drugs and smoking. Pesticides on non-organic fruit and vegetables also cause free radical damage within the body, as do toxins in our air.

There are some obvious answers to this problem: avoid processed foods, avoid alcohol, don't smoke, don't take drugs, avoid highly polluted environments and eat organic fruit and vegetables as often as you can (and wash thoroughly or peel those that aren't organic before you eat them). However, we can also minimise the rate of free radical damage in our body, and so slow down the ageing of our cells, by increasing our intake of nature's own antidotes to oxidative stress (another name for free radical damage) – namely, antioxidants. These heroes of the nutrient world travel around the body finding free radicals and generously handing over an electron to stabilise or neutralise them, thereby slowing down the ageing of our cells. This includes protecting the quality of the cells that make up sperm in men and especially the cells that make up the developing eggs within a woman's ovarian follicles.

For this reason, all couples over the age of 35 should boost the levels of antioxidants in their diet, which means seeking out foods that are rich in vitamins A, C and E (see page 67), as well as the minerals zinc and selenium.

Co-enzyme Q10 (co-Q10)

Studies show that the health of a woman's eggs may be particularly sensitive to levels of the enzyme co-Q10 in her body, which we both manufacture within our body and derive from our diet. Levels of co-Q10 lower as a natural side effect of the ageing process, which means that increasing dietary sources of this important nutrient can potentially have a significant impact on egg health. Oily fish, organ meats, pork, beef and chicken are all good sources, but also talk to your nutritionist about supplementation.

For men, early evidence indicates that co-Q10 supports sperm health, improving quantity and motility.

Low ovarian reserve

If you're over the age of 35 and your antral follicle count and anti-mullerian hormone test (see pages 12–13) have indicated that you have low ovarian reserve, don't despair. Instead, work on improving the quality of the eggs you do have by increasing your antioxidant intake and increasing levels of co-Q10, folic acid and inositol in your diet and through supplementation.

NOURISHING YOUR SPERM

Men manufacture sperm all the time, which means sperm production constantly draws from their nutritional intake and lifestyle influences. The food a man eats can influence:

* the total number of sperm cells produced (sperm count)
* their physical attributes (morphology)
* their ability to move properly once ejaculated (motility)
* the integrity of their DNA

These four elements make up overall sperm quality (see pages 82–3).

THE HUMAN SPERM

It's worth noting that the human sperm is one of the smallest human cells of all – 20 to 40 times smaller than a woman's egg – but it contains half the genetic information it takes to make a baby. It is a microscopic miracle of life. Understanding its make-up can help us understand which nutrients boost sperm quality.

The sperm is made up of three primary sections: the head, the midpiece and the tail. Let's start from the bottom up. The tail is what the sperm needs for propulsion, which occurs as a result of fine threads of tissue, called flagellum, that make a whip-like motion by sliding up and down against each other, driving the sperm forward. In order to do this, the sperm tail needs energy, which it gets from mitochondria that exist in spiral formation inside the midpiece. In fact, the midpiece is almost entirely made up of mitochondria. This leaves us with the head and it's here in the nucleus of this microscopic human cell that we find the man's 23 chromosomes, housing his DNA contribution to any potential baby. The nucleus is surrounded by a cell membrane that contains enzymes that help break down the outer membrane of the egg so that the sperm can penetrate it.

What do we mean by 'abnormal' sperm?

There are millions of sperm in every ejaculation, so it's perfectly expected that every semen sample will have a high number of abnormal forms. In fact, we look for only 4 per cent 'normality' in every semen sample. Looked at another way, a normal semen sample might have up to 96 per cent 'abnormal' sperm – that is 96 per cent of sperm might have an imperfectly shaped head or midpiece, or a problem with the tail, for example.

IMPROVING THE QUALITY OF YOUR SPERM

Amino acids, fatty acids and antioxidants are the three most important nutrient groups for sperm health, which broadly means that a diet of high-protein meat, fish and pulses, as well as nuts and seeds, and a rainbow of fruit and vegetables will provide the basics of the nutrients a man needs.

Within that broad range, certain foods provide specific nutrients especially valuable for sperm health. Diet and supplements can help to provide the right nutrition, including antioxidants to protect the sperm, energy and protein to provide the building blocks of life. Listed below are the nutrients it's especially important to boost in your diet and some examples of their food sources:

* **Arginine**
  This amino acid helps ensure good sperm morphology, reducing the numbers of abnormal sperm present in a semen sample. Arginine is found in protein-rich foods (especially in pork, beef, chicken, tuna and salmon, and in tinned anchovies).

* **Carnitine**
  This compound is a significant energy source for the mitochondrial cells within the sperm. It has been shown to increase sperm count, improve motility and straight-swimming ability. Red meat is a particularly good source of carnitine, as well as fish, poultry and milk. The body also synthesises carnitine from two amino acids: lysine and methionine. These are present in high-protein foods, such as eggs and meats. Pulses are also a good source of lysine and cereal grains of methionine.

* **Vitamin C and co-enzyme Q10**
  These antioxidants are known to improve sperm count, motility and morphology. Food sources of vitamin C include colourful fruit and vegetables. Co-enzyme Q10-rich foods include shellfish, pork, chicken, beef, sardines, mackerel and some nuts.

* **Vitamin E**
  Another antioxidant vitamin, vitamin E is known to reduce levels of chromosomal damage within the sperm and improve the sperm's ability to penetrate the egg membrane. Food sources are nuts and seeds (particularly sunflower seeds) and leafy green vegetables.

* **Zinc**
  An antioxidant mineral, zinc has long been thought to improve sperm count – you'll probably have come across advice that says men should eat oysters and prawns to boost sperm production! Nuts and seeds, pulses and turkey are also good sources.

* **Selenium**

  Another antioxidant, selenium in combination with N-acetylcysteine (NAC), a modified amino acid, is known to improve sperm motility, while NAC alone may also improve sperm count. Brazil nuts, wholegrain rice and leafy greens have higher levels of selenium than other foods. Selenium in combination with vitamin E has also been shown to help with motility and sperm quality.

* **Lycopene**

  Yet another antioxidant, lycopene is the compound that gives colour to foods such as tomatoes, red peppers and other red vegetables and fruits. Sperm seem to thrive on a diet rich in lycopene, increasing their quality and quantity.

* **Glutathione**

  This is an important antioxidant. We naturally produce glutathione and can increase levels by taking a supplement of NAC. Glutathione is also present in small amounts in some foods including asparagus, potato, leafy green vegetables, squash and grapefruit – among myriad other colourful fruit and vegetables. Like other antioxidants, it helps to protect the sperm against damage from free radicals, which means improving sperm morphology and motility overall.

* **Vitamin D**

  Vitamin D deficiency is linked to male infertility so make sure your levels are optimal. Sunlight and oily fish are both good sources.

* **Omega-3 fatty acids**

  DHA omega-3 is important to modulate the immune system and help with inflammation in the body. It regulates hormones and protects cell membranes. In addition, omega-3 fatty acids help to improve sperm count as well as sperm morphology and motility.

For men, good exercise levels may be an important factor in improving sperm count. One recent study of more than 200 men showed that those who exercised most had significantly improved sperm quantity per millilitre of semen compared with those who exercised least. The study was small and the researchers are careful to point out that we need more research to prove a link between exercise levels and sperm count (interestingly, motility and morphology seemed unaffected), but the foundation for a basic belief that exercising is good for a man's sperm production is there.

RECIPES FOR EGG HEALTH

Lime and Avocado Smoothie

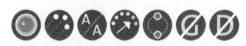

Thick and creamy thanks to the addition of avocado and coconut milk, this dairy-free smoothie is rich in healthy fats and inositol to support egg development. Use the zest and juice of the lime in the smoothie, which are rich in antioxidants including limonoids and vitamin C, known for their cell protective properties and alkalising benefits.

Preparation time: 5 minutes
Serves 2

INGREDIENTS

- 1 medium avocado, chopped
- a handful of spinach or other leafy greens
- juice and zest of 1 lime
- 1 tsp minced ginger
- 300 ml coconut milk
- 1 tsp coconut oil
- 1 chopped and frozen banana

PER SERVING	
Calories	185 kcal
Protein	2.4 g
Total Fat	12 g
Saturates	3.7 g
Carbohydrates	16.8 g
Sugar	15.6 g

Place all the ingredients together in a blender and process until smooth and creamy.

Health benefits

Don't be afraid to use fats in your smoothies. The right types of fat are essential for healthy pregnancy. Coconut oil is rich in medium-chain triglycerides (MCTs) which the body can preferentially use as a fuel source. Adding a teaspoonful to a smoothie is a great way to boost flagging energy levels and provide valuable anti-inflammatory fats.

Coconut Porridge with Berry and Cardamom Compote and Bee Pollen Sprinkle

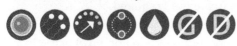

This is a deliciously warming breakfast option. The addition of tahini creates a wonderful creamy texture as well as plenty of calcium, zinc and a dose of healthy fats. Berries are packed with antioxidants and vitamin C to help protect egg and sperm from free radical damage. For an additional protein boost stir in a spoonful of protein powder at the end of cooking. Bee pollen has long been known as a fertility-boosting food. Rich in enzymes, amino acids, vitamins and minerals it is a restorative tonic for both men and women.

Preparation time: 10 minutes
Cooking time: 15 minutes
Serves 2

INGREDIENTS

For the berry and cardamom compote:
- 200 g mixed berries, fresh or frozen
- juice of ½ lemon
- 1 tsp xylitol (optional)
- 2 tsp cornflour
- seeds from 6 cardamom pods, crushed

PER SERVING	
Calories	326 kcal
Protein	18.8 g
Total Fat	8.9 g
Saturates	1 g
Carbohydrates	43 g
Sugar	12.8 g

For the porridge:
- 70 g porridge or gluten-free oats
- 200 ml coconut milk or coconut cream
- 1 tbsp tahini
- 1 scoop or 30 g plain or vanilla protein powder (optional)
- 2 tsp bee pollen

To make the compote, place the berries, lemon juice and xylitol, if using, in a pan along with two tablespoons of water. Cover and simmer gently over a low heat for 2–3 minutes until the berries have softened. Add a little extra water if needed. Mix the cornflour with two tablespoons of water to form a smooth paste. Add to the pan with the cardamom seeds and stir for 1–2 minutes until the mixture thickens. Set aside. The compote can be made ahead of time and kept in the fridge until required.

To make the porridge, place the oats, coconut milk and 400 ml of water in a saucepan and allow it to cook gently for about 10 minutes, until the liquid has all been absorbed and the porridge is thick. Stir in the tahini and protein powder if, using.

Spoon the porridge into bowls and top with the berry compote and a sprinkling of bee pollen.

Roasted Squash Soup with Chipotle Cream

Butternut squash is a delicious starchy vegetable loaded with antioxidants to help protect eggs and sperm from free radical damage. Roasting the squash produces a rich, sweet caramel flavour and, when blended, creates a wonderful creamy texture. If you cannot find tinned chipotle peppers, you can use a pinch of dried smoked chilli flakes instead.

Preparation time: 15 minutes
Cooking time: 45 minutes
Serves 2

INGREDIENTS

- 500 g butternut squash, cubed
- 1 tbsp olive oil
- 1 tbsp coconut oil
- ½ tsp chopped tinned chipotle peppers in adobo sauce
- ½ onion, chopped
- 1 carrot, chopped and peeled
- 1 garlic clove, crushed
- 600 ml vegetable or chicken stock
- sea salt and black pepper

PER SERVING	
Calories	258 kcal
Protein	6.1 g
Total Fat	14.2 g
Saturates	7.6 g
Carbohydrates	26.4 g
Sugar	17 g

For the chipotle cream:

- 3 tbsp natural yoghurt or kefir
- pinch of smoked chilli flakes or ½ tsp chopped tinned chipotle peppers or to taste

---

Preheat the oven to 180°C (gas mark 4). Place the butternut squash on a baking tray and drizzle with the olive oil. Season with salt and pepper. Bake in the oven for 20–30 minutes until golden. Set aside.

In a large pan heat the coconut oil and add the chipotle peppers, onion, carrot and garlic. Sauté for 5 minutes, then pour over the stock. Add the roasted butternut squash and simmer for 10 minutes. Purée the soup in a food processor or blender, or use an immersion hand blender.

For the chipotle cream, mix together the yoghurt and dried chilli or chopped chipotle pepper and season with salt and pepper.

Ladle the soup into bowls then swirl in a spoonful of the chipotle cream to serve.

Roasted Root Vegetable, Tomato and Lentil Salad with Lemon Tahini Dressing

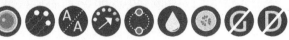

Tahini paste is made from ground sesame seeds. It's a good source of methionine, an amino acid which aids in liver detoxification. Tahini is also rich in minerals such as phosphorus, lecithin, magnesium, potassium and iron and is a great source of protein and healthy fats to support egg production and sperm health. Roasted root vegetables make a substantial warm salad that is equally delicious served cold. The tahini dressing can be prepared ahead of time and stored in the fridge for several days. Use it to dress a range of salads or drizzle over steamed vegetables.

Preparation time: 15 minutes
Cooking time: 42 minutes
Serves 2

INGREDIENTS

- 1 sweet potato, diced
- 1 beetroot, diced
- 1 carrot, peeled and diced
- 1 parsnip, peeled and diced
- 1 red onion, cut into thick wedges
- 1 tbsp olive oil
- 1 tsp za'atar
- 1 tsp coconut oil
- 12 cherry tomatoes, halved
- 30 g pine nuts
- 200 g cooked puy lentils, rinsed and drained
- sea salt and black pepper

For the tahini dressing:
- 4 tsp tahini
- 2 tbsp lemon juice
- 1 tsp honey
- pinch of za'atar

PER SERVING	
Calories	564 kcal
Protein	17.9 g
Total Fat	27.3 g
Saturates	4.3 g
Carbohydrates	61.5 g
Sugar	22.6 g

Preheat the oven to 200°C (gas mark 6).

Place the sweet potato, beetroot, carrot, parsnip and onion on a baking tray. Drizzle over the oil and za'atar and season well. Toss to coat.

Bake in the oven for 30–40 minutes until the vegetables are golden and tender.

Heat the coconut oil in a frying pan. Add the cherry tomatoes, pine nuts and lentils and sauté gently for 1–2 minutes to soften the tomatoes.

To make the tahini dressing, place the tahini in a bowl and whisk in three tablespoons of water, along with the lemon juice, honey and za'atar. Season to taste.

Place the vegetables on a platter and spoon over the lentil and tomato mixture. Drizzle over the dressing to serve.

Chermoula-baked Salmon

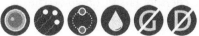

This fish dish is inspired by the flavours of North African cooking. It is a great source of omega-3 fats, which are essential for the health of eggs and sperm and for keeping inflammation in check. If you can marinate the fish overnight this will enhance its flavour and the sauce keeps the salmon wonderfully moist when cooked.

Preparation time: 10 minutes
Marinating time: 1–2 hours or overnight
Cooking time: 12 minutes
Serves 2

INGREDIENTS

For the chermoula:
- a handful of fresh coriander leaves
- a handful of fresh flat-leaf parsley
- a handful of fresh mint leaves
- 2 garlic cloves, chopped
- 1 tsp ground cumin
- 1 tsp ground coriander
- ½ tsp paprika
- 1 tsp harissa paste
- 2 tbsp lemon juice
- 4 tbsp olive oil
- sea salt and black pepper

For the salmon:
- 2 salmon fillets, about 120 g each, boneless and skinless

PER SERVING	
Calories	393 kcal
Protein	25.8 g
Total Fat	32 g
Saturates	5 g
Carbohydrates	0.9 g
Sugar	0.4 g

Line a baking tray with baking parchment.

To make the chermoula, place all the ingredients, except the salt and pepper, in a food processor and process to form a thick paste. Season with salt and pepper.

Season the skinned side of each salmon fillet with salt and pepper and then spread with some of the chermoula. Place chermoula-side down on the baking tray, then spread the other side with the remaining chermoula.

Cover the tray tightly with tin foil and marinate in the fridge for 1–2 hours or overnight, if possible.

When ready to cook, preheat the oven to 180°C (gas mark 4).

Bake the fish, still covered, in the oven for 10–12 minutes until cooked through.

Remove the salmon from the oven and discard the foil. Place the salmon on plates, spoon over the cooking juices from the baking tray and serve. Accompany with steamed vegetables or salad and sweet potato chips or wholegrain rice.

RECIPES FOR SPERM HEALTH

Virgin Bloody Mary

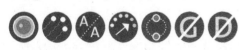

This energising, hydrating juice is rich in lycopene and is ideal for preparing the body for IVF. Lycopene is especially important for improving sperm health: a low intake of lycopene in the diet is associated with poor semen quality and male infertility.

Preparation time: 5 minutes
Serves 2

INGREDIENTS

- 6 medium-sized ripe tomatoes
- 2 celery sticks
- ½ cucumber
- 1 lime, peeled
- 3–4 dashes of Worcestershire sauce, to taste
- 3–4 dashes of Tabasco sauce, to taste
- ½ tsp baobab powder
- ½ tsp acai powder
- pinch of sea salt
- small slice of fresh horseradish (optional)
- crushed ice, to serve

PER SERVING	
Calories	50 kcal
Protein	2 g
Total Fat	1.2 g
Saturates	0.2 g
Carbohydrates	7.3 g
Sugar	6.9 g

Put the tomatoes, celery, cucumber and lime through a juicer. Stir in the remaining ingredients and serve with crushed ice.

Health benefits

The addition of superfoods like baobab and acai powder will give your juice a vitamin C boost.. Baobab contains six times the vitamin C content of oranges and is an excellent source of soluble fibre and to maintain healthy gut flora. Acai berry is renowned for its high antioxidant properties to help protect tissues and organs from oxidative damage which may lead to poor sperm health and quality.

Cranberry and Walnut Granola Cluster

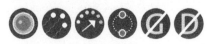

This delicious crunchy cereal is perfect for breakfast or as a healthy snack. Walnuts are rich in omega-3 fats and vitamin E, shown to be important for sperm quality and promoting endometrial health. The combination of nuts, seeds and oats in this recipe provides plenty of protein and energising B vitamins and magnesium. The granola clusters can be stored in an airtight container for up to two weeks in the fridge.

Preparation time: 10 minutes
Cooking time: 30 minutes
Makes 10 servings

INGREDIENTS

- 100 g almonds
- 100 g walnuts
- 100 g porridge or gluten-free oats
- 30 g protein powder
- 75 g dried cranberries
- 50 g pumpkin seeds
- 50 g sunflower seeds
- 30 g desiccated coconut
- 1 tsp cinnamon
- 30 g honey, yacon syrup, coconut syrup or maple syrup
- 30 g coconut oil, melted
- 1 tsp vanilla extract

PER SERVING	
Calories	312 kcal
Protein	23 g
Total Fat	23 g
Saturates	6.1 g
Carbohydrates	16.4 g
Sugar	8.5 g

Preheat the oven to 150°C (gas mark 3). Grease and line a baking tray with baking parchment.

Place the almonds in a food processor and process to a fine powder. Remove and place in a large bowl.

Place the walnuts and oats in the food processor and process to break up into fine pieces. Place into the bowl with the almonds. Add the remaining ingredients and mix thoroughly. If the mixture seems too dry add a splash of water.

Spread the mixture out on to the baking tray and press down to compact the mixture – this will help it to form clusters. Bake for 20–30 minutes, stirring once during cooking, until golden and cooked through.

Remove from the oven and allow to cool on the tray, then break the mixture into clusters. Serve with whole milk or almond milk and top with fresh berries.

Roasted Tomato, Tortilla and Chicken Soup

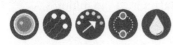

This warming soup is packed with antioxidants and protein. Cooking tomatoes actually enables you to absorb more lycopene – a potent compound shown to be important for sperm health.

Preparation time: 15 minutes
Cooking time: 23 minutes
Serves 2

INGREDIENTS

- 6 plum tomatoes, quartered
- ½ red onion, cut into large chunks
- 1 garlic clove
- 1 tbsp olive oil
- 1 tbsp coconut oil
- 1 carrot, finely chopped and peeled
- ½ tsp chilli powder
- ½ tsp ground cumin
- 350 ml chicken stock
- 1 tsp tomato purée
- 100 g cooked sweetcorn
- 250 g cooked chicken breast, shredded
- 1 tbsp fresh lime juice
- 1 flour tortilla, grilled and cut into thin strips
- 30 g Cheddar, grated
- 1 tbsp fresh coriander leaves, chopped
- sea salt and black pepper

PER SERVING	
Calories	472 kcal
Protein	48.6 g
Total Fat	17.2 g
Saturates	6.2 g
Carbohydrates	30.4 g
Sugar	14.4 g

Preheat the grill to high. Place the tomatoes, onion and garlic on a baking tray. Toss in the olive oil and season. Grill for 10–15 minutes until the tomatoes are soft and lightly golden. Place the tomato mixture into a blender and process to form a chunky purée.

Heat the coconut oil in a large pan and add the carrot, chilli powder and cumin. Sauté briefly for 2–3 minutes. Add the chicken stock and tomato purée and simmer for 5 minutes. Stir in the sweetcorn, shredded chicken and lime juice and cook for a further 5 minutes. Stir in most of the tortilla strips, saving a few strips to garnish.

Ladle the soup into bowls and scatter over a little cheese, the remaining tortilla strips and some coriander leaves to serve.

Garlic Baked Chicken with Romesco Sauce

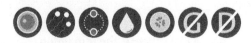

This recipe is very quick to prepare making it perfect for when time is short. If possible, marinate the chicken overnight before baking. The romesco sauce is packed with antioxidants, including lycopene known to support sperm heath. Garlic is a wonderful anti-inflammatory spice and is ideal for supporting detoxification pathways. This recipe is delicious served with steamed broccoli and green beans.

Preparation time: 15 minutes
Marinating time: 1–2 hours or overnight
Cooking time: 40 minutes
Serves 2

INGREDIENTS

- 1 tbsp olive oil
- 1 tsp honey
- ½ tsp smoked paprika
- pinch of chilli flakes
- 2 garlic cloves, crushed
- 4 chicken thigh fillets, about 100 g each, boneless, skin on
- 1 lemon, quartered
- ½ red onion, cut into wedges
- sea salt and black pepper
- a little chopped fresh parsley, to garnish

For the romesco sauce:

- 10 cherry tomatoes
- 2 garlic cloves
- 2 tbsp olive oil
- 1 roasted red pepper, from a jar, drained
- 60 g flaked toasted almonds
- 1 tsp red wine vinegar
- ¼ tsp smoked paprika
- pinch of cayenne pepper

PER SERVING	
Calories	487 kcal
Protein	33.8 g
Total Fat	34.3 g
Saturates	4.4 g
Carbohydrates	10.6 g
Sugar	8.7 g

In a small bowl whisk together the oil, honey, spices and garlic. Season with salt and pepper.

Place the chicken in a small roasting dish with the lemon and red onion and pour over the oil mixture. Coat thoroughly. Cover the dish tightly with cling film and marinate in the fridge for 1–2 hours or overnight, if possible.

Preheat the grill to medium and the oven to 190°C (gas mark 5).

To make the romesco sauce, place the tomatoes on a baking tray with the garlic cloves. Drizzle over a little of the olive oil and grill for 5–10 minutes until the tomatoes are lightly golden and have softened.

Place the tomatoes and the remaining ingredients for the sauce into a blender and process until smooth. Add a dash of water if needed to create a thick sauce.

Remove the chicken from the fridge and roast in the oven for 25–30 minutes or until the chicken is cooked through and golden. Serve the chicken with the romesco sauce and a sprinkling of parsley.

Fish Tagine with Green Olives and Preserved Lemon

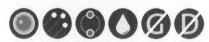

Packed with selenium and zinc to support the production of healthy sperm, this is a mild, mellow tagine with a refreshing tangy sauce thanks to the addition of preserved lemon and salty olives. Unlike meat tagines, this takes much less time to cook making it an easy after work dish.

Preparation time: 15 minutes
Cooking time: 27 minutes
Serves 2

INGREDIENTS

- 1 tbsp coconut oil
- ½ onion, finely sliced
- ½ garlic clove, chopped
- 1 tsp tomato purée
- ½ tsp turmeric powder
- ½ tsp ground cumin
- ½ tsp ground coriander
- 1 x 200 g tin chopped tomatoes
- 200 ml vegetable or chicken stock
- ½ x 400 g tin cooked chickpeas
- 1 tsp honey
- 8 okra, halved lengthways
- 1 carrot, diced and peeled
- 4 ready-to-eat apricots, chopped
- 1 preserved lemon, skin only, chopped
- 6 green olives, pitted
- 100 g quinoa, rinsed
- 2 firm white skinless fish fillets (for example, cod or haddock)
- 100 g raw peeled prawns
- fresh coriander leaves

PER SERVING	
Calories	356 kcal
Protein	42 g
Total Fat	10.2 g
Saturates	4.7 g
Carbohydrates	24 g
Sugar	14.1 g

Heat the coconut oil in a large pan and sauté the onion and garlic for 5 minutes until softened but not coloured.

Stir in the tomato purée and spices and cook for a further minute. Add the chopped tomatoes, stock, chickpeas, honey, okra, carrot, apricots, lemon and olives. Bring to a simmer and cook for 10–15 minutes until the vegetables are cooked.

Meanwhile, drain and place the quinoa in a separate pan with 400 ml of water. Bring to the boil then reduce the heat to very low, cover the pan and simmer for 15 minutes until cooked. Turn off the heat and leave the quinoa in the pan with the lid on while you finish the tagine.

Add the fish fillets and prawns to the tomato sauce and gently push them down so they are covered. Allow the fish to cook in the sauce over a very gentle heat, with the pan covered, for 5–7 minutes until the fish and prawns are cooked through.

Scatter over the coriander and serve with the quinoa.

Carrot Cake Pudding with Coconut Cream

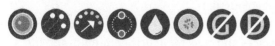

This raw carrot cake pudding is creamy and packed with protein and healthy fats. Carrots are a great source of antioxidants, known as carotenoids, which have been shown to improve sperm quality and motility. Antioxidants help to neutralise free radicals – destructive groups of atoms that are a by-product of metabolism and can damage cell membranes and DNA.

Preparation time: 15 minutes
Cooking time: 18 minutes
Serves 4

INGREDIENTS

For the carrot cake:
- 100 g soft dates, pitted
- 150 g carrot, finely grated
- 100 g pecans, ground in a food processor
- 30 g raisins
- ½ tsp mixed spice
- ½ tsp ground cinnamon
- 1 tbsp vanilla extract
- zest of 1 orange
- 30 g desiccated coconut

For the coconut cream:
- 50 g desiccated coconut
- 4 tbsp coconut cream or full-fat coconut milk
- juice and zest of 1 orange
- a little orange zest, to garnish

PER SERVING	
Calories	452 kcal
Protein	5.3 g
Total Fat	35.3 g
Saturates	16.7 g
Carbohydrates	28.1 g
Sugar	28.1 g

Place the dates in 100 ml of water and allow to soak for 15 minutes. Purée the dates with the soaking water in a blender or food processor to form a thick paste. Add the remaining ingredients for the cake to the food processor and blend briefly to combine but leaving plenty of texture.

For the coconut cream, simply place the ingredients in a blender and process until smooth and thick. Add a little more coconut cream if needed: it should be a similar consistency to thick Greek yoghurt.

Divide the carrot cake mixture between four small glasses. Top with half of the coconut cream and repeat the layering finishing with the cream. Decorate with a little additional orange zest if desired. Chill in the fridge until required.

CHAPTER ELEVEN

Nourishing Your Digestive System

All the good advice in the world about the foods you should eat to optimise your chances of having a baby is undermined if you don't have good gut health. Nourishing your digestive system and giving it a helping hand in terms of how and when you eat, are just as important. I would even go so far as to say that your gut health is the cornerstone of your whole well-being.

Poor gut health can trigger inflammation in your body and increase levels of free radicals (see pages 173 and 79 respectively), both of which will damage eggs and sperm. Using your diet to improve your gut health, looking at anti-inflammatory nutritional choices and ways in which you can use diet to modulate your immune system will pay dividends in terms of your ability to have a baby.

No amount of nutritional goodness is worthwhile if your gut itself – that is, your intestines and your colon, your gastrointestinal tract – is in poor working order. The ability of your gut lining to absorb nutrients, the proper release of enzymes to break down your food and your gut's ability to move efficiently to pass waste along its length are all important aspects of good intestinal health.

RECOGNISING THE SIGNS OF POOR GUT HEALTH

If you suffer from constipation, irritable bowel syndrome (IBS), bloating, diarrhoea or indigestion on a regular basis, you almost certainly have poor gut health. The knock-on effect is that you'll feel lethargic, tired and 'full'. You'll probably suffer mood swings and, in particular, irritability. You may break out in acne or start to suffer allergies or intolerances to certain foods. Internally, what's going on in your gut will impact your immune system, cause inflammation in your body and ultimately affect the health of your gut lining.

GUT AGGRAVATORS

Processed foods (including junk foods) and foods high in refined sugar place a strain on your digestive system, promoting the growth of pathogenic bacteria and yeast which can disrupt digestion, promote inflammation and contribute to gut barrier damage. High-gluten foods (gluten is found in barley, rye and wheat and is the sticky substance in starchy foods such as bread and pasta), as well as alcohol and caffeine are also aggravating for the intestine.

Furthermore, stress can disrupt the levels of beneficial bacteria in the gut and promote inflammation.

IMPROVING GUT HEALTH

It's so important to enhance your gut health to optimise the chances of IVF working for you as poor digestion can affect your odds of IVF success. Here are my top tips for good gut health:

* Don't eat late in the evening. Allow three hours after eating before going to bed to support digestion.
* Avoid high-sugar foods and drinks, including fruit juices and all-fruit smoothies, which can feed pathogenic bacteria and yeasts in the digestive tract promoting dysbiosis (imbalance of beneficial bacteria). This can lead to bloating and damage to the gut lining.
* Increase your intake of fermented foods which can naturally increase levels of beneficial bacteria in the gut. Examples include probiotic yoghurts, kefir, nattō, tempeh, sauerkraut, kimchi and kombucha.
* Naturally increase digestive secretions to improve your digestion. Drink lemon juice in warm water in the morning to kick-start digestion and include bitter greens like watercress, rocket and dandelion in your meals. Other foods like papaya and pineapple contain digestive enzymes which can promote digestion and lower inflammation.
* Reduce inflammation and repair the wall of the intestine by eating foods that are rich in antioxidant vitamins (particularly vitamins A, C and E; see pages 67–70), as well as omega-3 fatty acids (in fish, nuts and seeds) and glutamine (present in protein foods, such as seafood, meat, poultry and pulses). Spices such as turmeric are also known for their anti-inflammatory benefits.
* Restore the acid–alkaline balance in the gut by eating more alkaline-rich foods (see pages 162–5), including kale and other leafy green vegetables, and limit consumption of refined grains and processed meats.

Improving digestion

Certain foods are good at improving the process of digestion, too. Try including more of the following in your diet: cinnamon, turmeric, zinc-rich foods (leafy greens, seafood, turkey, pumpkin seeds), ginger, papaya, pineapple and bitter greens.

THE WAY YOU EAT

In Traditional Chinese Medicine, the way in which we eat and when we eat have a significant impact on digestive efficiency. Scientific studies bear out this ancient methodology. The Chinese believe that while you're eating you should eat; while you're drinking, you should drink; and while you're thinking, you should think. They believe that to try to do all three (or even a combination of two of the three) at once is to dilute the efficiency and effectiveness of each task. With this in mind, I recommend that all my clients consider how they eat and when.

Whenever you can (even if it's just at the weekends), follow the adage to breakfast like a king, lunch like a prince and dine like a pauper. This means eating your biggest and most nutrient-dense meal in the morning (ideally between 7 and 9 am when your stomach is ready for food after the period of fasting during sleep) and having your lightest meals in the evening (the Chinese believe that your stomach takes its rest between 7 and 9 pm and so doesn't want to be busy digesting). When this isn't practical, eat your daily intake of carbs mostly at breakfast and lunch, and make your evening meal carb-light and rich in protein (a piece of grilled, lean meat, for example, with a salad).

Concentrate on your meal – savour the food on the plate even before you take the first mouthful (digestion begins with the eyes, not the mouth). And turn off your phone, the television and your laptop! Eat mindfully, appreciating the sights and smells of your food; and talk to each other between mouthfuls so that you don't gulp down your food. Take time to chew – chewing signals to your gut that nutrients are on their way, stimulating your digestive juices. It also means you're less likely to overeat (each mouthful has time to hit your stomach before you're ready to swallow the next). You'll also learn to separate the flavours in your food, which will make you more sensitive to flavours that aren't good for you – salt and sugar among them – so you'll use them less in your cooking.

SPECIAL DIETS

Whether through choice (for example, being vegetarian or vegan) or as a result of food intolerance, allergy or another condition, not everyone who comes to see me in the clinic can eat every type of food. Part of our job is to give advice to those with special diets to ensure they also maximise nutritional intake to improve their chances of IVF success.

VEGETARIAN

Meat is a complete protein (see page 64), meaning that it contains all the essential building blocks (amino acids) the body needs to build and repair its cells. For vegetarians, however, eggs and dairy also provide important complete sources, as do quinoa, buckwheat, spirulina and chia seeds (however, as you don't eat seeds in large quantities, it's best not to think of them as a main source of protein). Furthermore, a varied diet that includes different types of beans, pulses, nuts and seeds will build up the bank of essential amino acids to ensure that vegetarians get everything they need for optimum health.

Iron may also be low in your diet, so it's important to eat plenty of leafy green vegetables, lentils and dried fruits, as well as a little blackstrap molasses. If you drink a glass of orange juice with iron-rich foods it will help your body with absorption. Vegetarian diets may also be lacking in the omega-3 fats DHA and EPA which are predominately found in oily fish. Therefore, you may wish to supplement to obtain these fatty acids.

VEGAN

Vegans do not consume any animal products including dairy and eggs and therefore it is important to include a variety of protein-rich alternatives in your diet to ensure you get all the essential amino acids your body needs. Beans, pulses, soya products, nuts, seeds and leafy green vegetables are all good sources. However, please be aware that although leafy greens can contribute some protein, they are not a main source: an 80 g portion of cooked kale contains only 3.7 g of protein, whereas 120 g of cooked chickpeas contains over 10 g.

Variety is key – as long as your plant-based diet is varied and broad, you should get all the nutrients you need. Calcium-rich plant foods must also be high on your shopping list: oranges, leafy green vegetables, fortified milk alternatives and tahini (sesame seed paste) are good sources. And don't forget the mighty avocado – a powerhouse of good fats, as well as plant protein. Iodine levels may be low so try to consume a couple of portions of sea vegetables each week and consider taking an omega-3 supplement sourced from algae. We have provided a number of healthy vegan recipes in this book to help you include all the vitamins and nutrients you need.

GLUTEN-FREE

If you suffer from coeliac disease (now affecting an estimated 1 in 100 people in the UK) or have a gluten intolerance, you will need to avoid wheat-, barley- and rye-based products. This means many everyday carbohydrate foods, including pasta, bread and most cereals, will not be suitable. However, carbohydrate is also present in many gluten-free foods, including quinoa, rice, sweet potato, buckwheat, amaranth, flaxseed, chia seeds and nut flours, which will also provide you with the fibre you need. Check out the recipes showing the gluten-free symbol for some ideas.

RECIPES FOR GUT HEALTH

Vitamin C Kefir Strawberry Shake

Kefir is a traditional fermented drink packed with beneficial bacteria. If you cannot tolerate dairy you can use coconut kefir in this recipe which is now widely available. Adding a spoonful of baobab is a great way to boost your intake of vitamin C, while the superberry powder provides a wealth of protective antioxidants.

Preparation time: 5 minutes
Serves 2

INGREDIENTS

- 200 g hulled strawberries, chopped
- 1 tsp goji berry or superberry food powder
- ½ tsp baobab powder
- 300 ml kefir or coconut kefir
- 2 tbsp gluten-free or regular porridge oats

PER SERVING	
Calories	190 kcal
Protein	7.5 g
Total Fat	7.2 g
Saturates	3.5 g
Carbohydrates	23.6 g
Sugar	13.2 g

Place all the ingredients in a blender and process until smooth.

Health benefits

Oats are a great source of slow-releasing carbohydrates and soluble fibre, which can help balance blood sugar levels and promote digestion and the growth of beneficial bacteria in the gut.

Beetroot and Apple Pickle

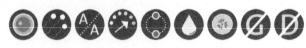

Making your own fermented vegetables is a great way to improve your digestive health and provide plenty of beneficial bacteria to support a healthy immune system and lower inflammation in the body. Try to include a small amount daily to balance your gut flora. This recipe uses a vegetable starter culture which is a preparation used to kick-start the fermentation process when culturing vegetables. These contain a broad spectrum of beneficial bacteria and produce consistent results to improve digestive health. They are readily available from health food shops and online suppliers. Try this fermented gut-healthy pickle served with burgers or spooned over salads. It also works well with fish, eggs and lean meats.

Preparation time: 15 minutes
Fermenting time: 2 weeks
Makes 1 x 1 litre jar
Serves 8

INGREDIENTS

- 1 litre glass preserving jar with lid, sterilised

- 3 carrots
- 2 beetroots
- 2 apples, cored and finely chopped
- ½ red onion, finely chopped
- 4 cloves
- 2 star anise
- 1 tbsp juniper berries
- 30 g goji berries
- 1 tbsp sea salt
- 2 tbsp warm water
- 1 sachet vegetable starter culture

PER SERVING	
Calories	46 kcal
Protein	0.8 g
Total Fat	0.4 g
Saturates	0.1 g
Carbohydrates	9.9 g
Sugar	9.3 g

Wash and sterilise the preserving jar in a hot rinse cycle in the dishwasher or use very hot water.

Grate the carrot and beetroot using a coarse grater – you can use a food processor attachment to do this or grate by hand. Place the vegetables in a large bowl. Add the apple, red onion, spices and goji berries.

Dissolve the salt in the warm water, then pour into the bowl, massaging the salt into the mixture with your hands.

Dissolve the starter culture in water according to the packet instructions. (The amount of water may vary depending on the brand used: typically it is 125 ml.) Add the culture to the bowl.

Fill the sterilised preserving jar with the mixture, pressing down well with a large spoon to remove any air pockets. Pour in any remaining water. The mixture should be completely submerged in the liquid. If not, add a little more water. Ideally leave about 2 cm of room free at the top of the jar as the vegetables can expand during fermentation.

Place a cabbage leaf on top of the mixture and add a small weight (for example, a small ramekin, tin or shot glass) on top to keep everything submerged. Clamp the jar tightly. Store the jar at room temperature (around 20°C) and ferment for 10–14 days.

Taste the mixture – it should taste tangy and slightly sour. Chill the jar in the fridge. Once opened, store in the fridge and use within 5–10 days.

Lamb Koftas with Herb Dip

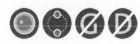

Including yoghurt regularly in your diet is an easy way to boost levels of beneficial bacteria to support digestive health and immune function. You can make this recipe dairy-free by replacing the yoghurt with coconut yoghurt or coconut kefir. This fabulous protein-packed dish is perfect for lunch with a simple mixed salad or accompanied by steamed vegetables and sweet potato chips for an evening meal.

Preparation time: 15 minutes
Cooking time: 15 minutes
Serves 2 (makes 4 skewers)

INGREDIENTS

For the lamb koftas:

- 1 tbsp pine nuts, toasted
- 2 tbsp fresh coriander leaves, chopped
- 1 tsp ground cumin
- 1 tsp ground coriander
- 1 tsp chopped red chilli
- ½ tsp turmeric powder
- zest and juice of 1 lime
- 250 g lean lamb mince
- sea salt and black pepper

For the herb dip:

- 100 g Greek-style yoghurt
- 1 tbsp fresh coriander leaves
- 1 tbsp fresh mint leaves, chopped

PER SERVING	
Calories	366 kcal
Protein	28.2 g
Total Fat	27.2 g
Saturates	11.5 g
Carbohydrates	2.9 g
Sugar	2.7 g

Preheat the oven to 200°C (gas mark 6). Grease and line a baking tray with baking parchment.

Place the pine nuts in a food processor and chop finely.

Place all the ingredients for the koftas, except the salt and pepper, in a large bowl and mix well with your hands so that the mixture sticks together. Season well. With damp hands, take a handful of the kofta mixture and shape into a long sausage shape around a metal skewer. Repeat with the remaining kebab mixture, using a new skewer each time.

Place the skewers on the baking tray and cook in the oven for 12–15 minutes, turning them halfway, until the lamb is golden brown and cooked through. Slide the koftas off the skewers and set aside.

For the herb dip, mix the ingredients together in a bowl, season to taste and set aside.

Serve the koftas topped with the herb dip.

Miso Glazed Cod with Sesame Seeds and Wilted Pak Choi

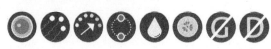

This is a classic Japanese fish dish: the fish is soaked in a salty-sweet miso marinade before cooking. Miso and tamari are both fermented products known for their digestive benefits. Serve this with Beetroot and Apple Pickle (see above) for a probiotic boost. You could double up on this recipe and serve leftovers with salad the following day for an easy lunch. Pak choi is a member of the cruciferous vegetable family making it valuable to support detoxification as well as being rich in egg-friendly nutrients, including vitamin A, B vitamins, folic acid, manganese and iron.

Preparation time: 15 minutes
Marinating time: 1–2 hours or overnight
Cooking time: 13 minutes
Serves 2

INGREDIENTS

For the miso marinade:

- 1 tbsp honey, maple syrup or yacon syrup
- 2 tbsp tamari soya sauce
- 2 tbsp white miso paste
- 2 tbsp mirin

For the cod:

- 2 cod fillets, about 120 g each, boneless, skin on
- 2 tbsp coconut oil
- 2 pak choi
- 1 garlic clove, crushed
- 1 tbsp sesame seeds, toasted
- 2 lemon wedges

For the dressing:

- 1 tbsp tahini
- 2 tsp tamari soya sauce
- 1 tsp xylitol
- 2 tsp rice vinegar

PER SERVING	
Calories	338 kcal
Protein	30.4 g
Total Fat	16.6 g
Saturates	8.8 g
Carbohydrates	16.1 g
Sugar	10.3 g

To make the marinade, whisk together the honey, tamari, miso paste and mirin in a small bowl.

Pat the cod fillets thoroughly dry with paper towels. Slather the fish with the miso marinade and place in a shallow dish. Cover the dish tightly with cling film and marinate in the fridge for 1–2 hours or overnight, if possible.

When ready to cook, preheat the oven to 200°C (gas mark 6).

Heat one tablespoon of the coconut oil in an ovenproof frying pan. Place the fish skin-side-up in the pan and cook until the bottom of the fish browns, about 3 minutes. Flip and continue cooking until the other side is browned, about 2–3 minutes. Transfer the pan to the oven and bake for 5–7 minutes, until the fish is opaque and cooked through.

While the fish is cooking, cut a thick slice from the pak choi root to separate the leaves. Rinse and drain the leaves. Heat the remaining coconut oil in a frying pan or wok and add the garlic and pak choi. Stir briefly to coat in the oil then place a lid on top and reduce the heat. Cook for 3–5 minutes, stirring occasionally, until the leaves have wilted.

To make the dressing, combine the tahini, tamari, xylitol and rice vinegar in a small bowl and whisk until smooth. Add a little water if needed to form a thick sauce. Drizzle over the pak choi and toss well.

Sprinkle the fish with the sesame seeds and serve with the pak choi and lemon wedges.

Acai Blueberry Ripple Ice Cream

Rich and creamy this quick ice cream is packed with superfoods to enhance fertility. Acai powder and blueberries are full of antioxidants to help protect sperm and eggs from free radical damage. The addition of kefir provides beneficial bacteria to support digestive health and lower inflammation. If kefir is not available use natural yoghurt instead. The ice cream can be stored in the freezer for up to three months.

Preparation time: 15 minutes
Cooking time: 18 minutes
Serves 4

INGREDIENTS

- 300 g blueberries, fresh or frozen
- 60 g xylitol
- juice of ½ lemon
- 200 ml coconut milk or whole milk
- 3 egg yolks
- 2 tbsp vanilla extract
- 100 g maple syrup, honey or coconut syrup
- 200 ml kefir, coconut kefir or natural yoghurt
- 1 tsp acai powder

PER SERVING	
Calories	197 kcal
Protein	2.9 g
Total Fat	5 g
Saturates	1.4 g
Carbohydrates	40.4 g
Sugar	24.2 g

Place the blueberries, xylitol and lemon juice in a pan with a splash of water. Simmer gently for 10 minutes or until the blueberries form a thick compote and the xylitol has dissolved. Set aside and allow to cool.

Place the milk in a separate pan and heat gently for about 2–3 minutes, stirring continuously. Take off the heat and set aside.

In a bowl whisk the egg yolks, vanilla extract and maple syrup together until the mixture is pale and fluffy. Keep whisking and gradually pour in the warm milk. Pour the mixture into a clean pan and cook gently, stirring all the time until the mixture begins to thicken. This may take about 5 minutes.

Take the pan off the heat and cool slightly. Blend in the kefir and acai powder. Pour into a jug, cover and place in the fridge to cool – this will take about an hour.

Once cooled, churn the mixture in an ice cream maker and, as it begins to thicken and freeze, pour in the blueberry compote and combine. Serve immediately.

Cherry and Apple Crisp

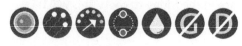

A warming and filling dessert, this is the ideal healthy comfort food. The cherries and apples are rich in polyphenols, potent antioxidants to protect the egg and sperm from damage. Polyphenols have also been shown to support the growth of beneficial bacteria in the gut and support digestive health.

Preparation time: 15 minutes
Cooking time: 23 minutes
Serves 4

INGREDIENTS

For the crumble topping:

- 125 g pecan halves
- 30 g desiccated coconut
- 1 tbsp honey or maple syrup
- 1 tbsp melted coconut oil
- ½ tsp vanilla extract

- 2 eating apples, cored and chopped
- 200 g frozen pitted cherries
- 1 tbsp honey or maple syrup

PER SERVING	
Calories	348 kcal
Protein	3.9 g
Total Fat	28.9 g
Saturates	7.7 g
Carbohydrates	17.8 g
Sugar	17.5 g

Preheat the oven to 180°C (gas mark 4).

To make the topping, place the pecan halves in a food processor and pulse briefly to chop. Add the remaining topping ingredients and pulse again to incorporate.

Place the apples, cherries and maple syrup in a pan and heat gently. Simmer for 2–3 minutes until the apples are beginning to soften.

Spoon the mixture into a small baking dish. Sprinkle over the crumble topping. Bake in the oven for 20 minutes until the crumble is lightly golden and the fruit is bubbling.

RECIPES FOR SPECIAL DIETS, ALLERGIES AND INTOLERANCES

Sweet Potato Protein Pancakes with Caramel Sauce

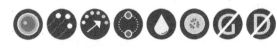

This is a delicious gluten-free protein-rich pancake recipe which is ideal for a weekend brunch or as a healthy snack. Sweet potatoes are packed with beta-carotene, vitamin C, B vitamins and manganese – all important for healthy eggs and protecting sperm quality. Sweet potatoes are also rich in soluble fibre helping to support healthy digestion and stabilising blood sugar levels. Adding a spoonful of protein powder to the batter is an easy way to increase your protein intake at breakfast. The caramel sauce is also delicious used as a dip with slices of fruit or simply poured over fruit salad. You can make the pancakes ahead of time and warm them up when needed. They are perfect served with Greek or coconut yoghurt and fresh berries.

Preparation time: 15 minutes
Cooking time: 6 minutes
Makes 4–6 pancakes
Serves 2

INGREDIENTS

For the caramel sauce:
- 8 dates (soaked for 10 minutes then drained and pitted)
- 2 tbsp lucuma powder, sifted
- 2 tbsp almond nut butter
- 1 tsp vanilla extract
- 100 ml whole, almond or coconut milk

For the pancakes:
- 150 g steamed sweet potato
- 50 g vanilla, plain or chocolate protein powder
- 2 eggs
- ½ tsp baking powder
- 1 tsp vanilla extract
- ½ tsp ground cinnamon
- 1 tbsp coconut oil, for cooking

PER SERVING	
Calories	531 kcal
Protein	32.3 g
Total Fat	21.4 g
Saturates	8.2 g
Carbohydrates	52.4 g
Sugar	24.9 g

To make the caramel sauce, place all the ingredients in a blender and process to form a thick sauce. Place in the fridge until required.

To make the pancakes, place all the ingredients, except the coconut oil, in a blender and process to form a thick batter.

Heat a little of the coconut oil in a frying pan until hot. Add spoonfuls of batter to the pan, spaced apart, and cook for 1–2 minutes until the pancakes are golden at the edges. Flip over and cook for a further minute. Remove and repeat with the remaining batter.

Place the pancakes on plates and serve with a little caramel sauce.

Turmeric Seeded Bread

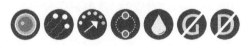

This is a protein-rich, gluten-free bread ideal for breakfast, as a healthy snack or as an accompaniment to soups and stews. This bread is full of protein and fibre from the nuts and seeds as well as omega-3 fatty acids, calcium and magnesium from the chia seeds. Adding a spoonful of turmeric helps create this fabulous anti-inflammatory bread and the addition of lucuma powder helps provide natural sweetness. Try toasting it and serving with scrambled eggs for a nourishing breakfast. You can store the bread in the fridge for three to five days or slice it and freeze for up to three months.

Preparation time: 15 minutes
Chilling time: 45 minutes
Makes 1 loaf (cuts into 8 slices)

INGREDIENTS

- 100 g mixed seeds (for example, sunflower, flaxseed and pumpkin)
- 1 tbsp chia seeds
- 1 tsp psyllium husks
- 200 g ground almonds
- 2 tsp turmeric powder
- 1 tbsp lucuma powder
- 1 tsp bicarbonate of soda
- 1 tsp baking powder
- 30 g coconut flour
- ½ tsp sea salt
- 1 tbsp coconut sugar or xylitol
- 6 eggs, beaten
- 1 tbsp apple cider vinegar
- 60 g coconut oil, melted

PER SERVING	
Calories	391 kcal
Protein	13.7 g
Total Fat	32.6 g
Saturates	10.2 g
Carbohydrates	10.1 g
Sugar	2.8 g

Preheat the oven to 160°C (gas mark 3). Grease and line a 2 lb loaf tin.

Place the dry ingredients in a food process or and pulse to combine.

Mix together the eggs and other wet ingredients then pour into the food processor. Process briefly to form a batter. Do not overprocess as you want to keep texture from the seeds.

Pour the batter into the lined loaf tin and bake in the oven for 45 minutes or until golden and a skewer inserted in the centre comes out clean.

Allow the bread to cool in the tin before turning out. Slice and serve.

Sun-dried Tomato Gluten-free Crackers

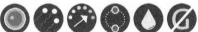

These delicious gluten-free crackers are packed with soluble fibre and protein to maintain healthy blood sugar levels and digestive health. They are ideal as a snack spread with nut butter, avocado or Speedy Smoked Mackerel Pâté (see page 213). The crackers can be stored in an airtight container for up to one week.

Preparation time: 15 minutes
Cooking time: 15 minutes
Makes 12 crackers

INGREDIENTS

- 15 g ground flaxseed
- 150 g gluten-free oats
- 75 g almond flour
- 75 g arrowroot flour
- ½ teaspoon sea salt
- ½ teaspoon bicarbonate of soda
- ½ tsp baking powder
- 60 g unsalted butter or coconut oil, melted
- 3 tbsp whole or almond milk
- 2 tbsp maple syrup, honey or coconut syrup
- 60 g sun-dried tomatoes, finely chopped

PER CRACKER	
Calories	184 kcal
Protein	3.3 g
Total Fat	11.8 g
Saturates	3.4 g
Carbohydrates	16 g
Sugar	2.1 g

Preheat the oven to 180°C (gas mark 4). Line a large baking tray with baking parchment.

Place the flaxseed, oats, flours, salt and bicarbonate of soda in a food processor and process until fine. Add the remaining ingredients and process to form a soft dough.

Wrap the dough in cling film and place in the fridge for 30 minutes.

Roll out the dough between two sheets of baking parchment. Use a cookie cutter to cut out crackers and place on the baking tray.

Bake for 15 minutes or until lightly golden. Allow to cool on a wire rack.

Malaysian Mee Goreng

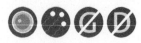

This Malay dish takes only a few minutes to cook once you have prepared your ingredients and is incredibly versatile – it's a great way to use up leftover vegetables from the fridge. This vegetarian version includes eggs, frozen peas and beans for protein. Peas and beans are an excellent food for developing good follicle quality for fertility. They are high in fibre, a good source of protein and are also rich in folic acid and iron to support fertility.

Preparation time: 15 minutes
Cooking time: 10 minutes
Serves 2

INGREDIENTS

- 150 g buckwheat or egg noodles
- 2 tbsp coconut oil
- ½ red onion, finely chopped
- 1 garlic clove, crushed
- 1 green chilli, deseeded and sliced
- 1 pak choi, chopped coarsely
- 50 g fresh or frozen shelled edamame beans
- 2 tsp sambal oelek (or other savoury chilli paste)
- 1 tbsp tamari soya sauce
- 1 tbsp Kecap Manis (sweet soya sauce)
- 2 tbsp tomato ketchup
- 50 g beansprouts
- 50 g frozen peas
- a handful of baby spinach leaves
- 2 eggs, beaten
- 2 lemon wedges

PER SERVING	
Calories	590 kcal
Protein	24.8 g
Total Fat	25.4 g
Saturates	11.5 g
Carbohydrates	65.7 g
Sugar	10.8 g

Cook the noodles in boiling water for 1–2 minutes only – they should still have a bite and not be too soft. Drain well.

Put a wok or large pan over the heat. Once hot, add the oil, then the onion and garlic and cook to soften for 1 minute. Add the green chilli, pak choi and edamame beans and let the pak choi wilt slightly, about 2 minutes.

Add the noodles, sambal oelek and all the sauces and toss carefully using tongs. Cook gently for 1–2 minutes. Add the beansprouts, frozen peas and spinach and cook for a further minute.

Make a well in the centre of the mixture and pour in the beaten egg. Let it cook for 1 minute then stir the egg into the noodles with a wooden spoon.

Spoon on to plates and serve with lemon wedges.

Jamaican Jerk Veggie Burgers with Carrot and Celeriac Slaw

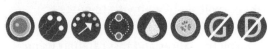

These vegetarian burgers, flavoured with a Jamaican-inspired spice paste, are wonderfully fragrant. The addition of beans provides plenty of protein and oats are rich in soluble fibre to help stabilise blood sugar levels and support digestive health. Celeriac is a great source of fibre to support detoxification and digestion and provides plenty of vitamin C and manganese for antioxidant support. The slaw is simple to make and can be kept in the fridge for two to three days.

Preparation time: 20 minutes
Cooking time: 10 minutes
Makes 4 burgers

INGREDIENTS

For the jerk paste:

- 2 spring onions chopped
- 1-cm piece of fresh ginger, chopped
- 3 garlic cloves, chopped
- ½ small onion, chopped
- 1 scotch bonnet chilli, deseeded and chopped
- 1 tbsp lime juice
- 2 tbsp tamari soya sauce
- 2 tbsp olive oil
- ½ tsp dried thyme
- 2 tsp coconut sugar or xylitol
- 1 tsp ground allspice

PER BURGER	
Calories	583 kcal
Protein	16.8 g
Total Fat	29.3 g
Saturates	5.4 g
Carbohydrates	63.8 g
Sugar	18 g

For the burgers:

- 1 x 400 g tin cooked red kidney beans, rinsed and drained
- 75 g rolled or gluten-free oats
- 1 egg, beaten
- sea salt and black pepper

For the slaw:

- 60 g Greek or coconut yoghurt
- 2 tbsp mayonnaise

- 1 tbsp lemon juice
  - 1 tbsp cider vinegar
  - 1 tsp honey
  - 100 g celeriac, peeled and grated
  - 1 carrot, peeled and grated
  - 1 apple, cored and grated
  - ¼ red onion, finely diced
  - 5 g fresh chopped mint leaves

Place the ingredients for the jerk paste in a food processor and process to form a thick paste. To make the burgers, add the beans, oats and egg and blend briefly to combine everything but keep some texture. Season with salt and pepper.

Divide the mixture into four, then wet your hands and shape into burgers. These can now be frozen if wished.

To make the slaw, in a small bowl whisk together the yoghurt, mayonnaise, lemon juice, vinegar and honey until smooth. Place the vegetables in a large bowl and pour over the dressing. Mix in the chopped mint and season to taste.

Preheat the grill to medium.

To cook the burgers, place them on a non-stick baking tray and grill for 5 minutes on each side until golden and crisp.

Serve the burgers topped with the slaw and accompany with a mixed salad or steamed vegetables.

> If you are cooking the burgers from frozen, bake at 200°C (gas mark 6) for 20–30 minutes until cooked through and lightly brown.

Kale Hemp Pesto with Courgette and Carrot Noodles

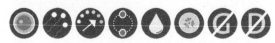

This version of pesto is packed with omega-3 fats and protein thanks to the addition of hemp seeds and kale. If you are preparing this as part of the two-week cleanse (see page 148), omit the dairy and use nutritional yeast flakes instead. Nutritional yeast flakes are readily available from health food shops or online and are a popular choice in vegan dishes. Packed with B vitamins, yeast flakes provide a cheesy, tangy flavour to dishes. If you don't have a spiraliser you can use a swivel potato peeler and make long ribbons instead.

Preparation time: 15 minutes
Serves 2

INGREDIENTS

For the pesto:

- 60 g hemp seeds, shelled
- 30 g pine nuts, toasted
- 2 garlic cloves, chopped
- 60 g kale, large stalks removed, chopped
- 15 g basil leaves
- 2 tbsp lemon juice
- 30 g Parmesan, grated or 2 tbsp nutritional yeast flakes
- 60 ml extra virgin olive oil, flaxseed oil or macadamia nut oil
- 100 g feta cheese, crumbled or ½ x 400 g tin cooked chickpeas
- sea salt and black pepper

For the noodles:

- 2 courgettes
- 2 carrots
- 4 basil leaves, torn
- 8 cherry tomatoes, halved

PER SERVING (WITH FETA)	
Calories	814 kcal
Protein	31.2 g
Total Fat	69.8 g
Saturates	15.9 g
Carbohydrates	15 g
Sugar	12.1 g

To make the pesto, put the hemp seeds, pine nuts, garlic, kale, basil and lemon juice in a food processor and whizz to a paste. Season to taste. Add the cheese or nutritional yeast flakes and gradually add enough oil to form a thick paste.

Using a sprialiser, create long noodles with the courgettes and carrots. Place in a large bowl with the basil leaves and cherry tomatoes. Stir through the pesto and top with feta cheese or chickpeas to serve.

Gluten-free Lemon Syrup Cake

A moist dessert cake, this is delicious served with yoghurt. Using xylitol helps keep the sugar content low and the addition of ground almonds boosts the protein content to help stabilise blood sugar levels. This will keep well in the fridge for three to four days and can be frozen for up to three months.

Preparation time: 15 minutes
Cooking time: 53 minutes
Makes 1 x 20-cm cake
Cuts into 10 slices

INGREDIENTS

For the cake:

- 200 g unsalted butter or coconut oil
- 100 g xylitol
- 3 large eggs
- 1 tbsp vanilla extract
- 1 tbsp lemon juice
- zest of 2 lemons
- 1 tsp baobab powder
- 200 g ground almonds
- 100 g fine polenta
- 1 tsp baking powder
- 1 tbsp lucuma powder (optional)

For the lemon syrup:

- juice of 2 lemons
- 3 tbsp xylitol

PER SLICE	
Calories	372 kcal
Protein	7 g
Total Fat	29.4 g
Saturates	11.8 g
Carbohydrates	25.5 g
Sugar	1.4 g

Preheat the oven to 160°C (gas mark 3). Grease and line a 20-cm springform cake tin with baking parchment.

To make the cake, place the butter in a food processor with the xylitol and beat until light and creamy.

Gradually beat in the eggs, vanilla extract, lemon juice and lemon zest. Slowly add the remaining ingredients and combine.

Spoon the batter into the cake tin. Bake for 40–50 minutes until the cake is golden or until a skewer inserted in the centre comes out clean.

Leave the cake to cool in the tin for 10 minutes then turn out.

To make the syrup, place the lemon juice and xylitol in a small saucepan and simmer gently to dissolve the xylitol. This should take about 3 minutes.

Prick the cake all over with a skewer, then pour over the syrup.

Cut into slices to serve.

Citrus Cashew Cream Tarts

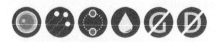

These refreshing little tarts are packed with healthy fats with the addition of nuts in the base and filling. Adding a spoonful of inositol powder is also another way of providing essential nutrients for egg health. Getting adequate amounts of vitamin C in your diet has been shown to help with male fertility: citrus fruits are a great source of vitamin C and protective antioxidants, and baobab fruit powder is exceptionally high in vitamin C. Once prepared, these tarts can be frozen for up to three months.

Preparation time: 20 minutes
Soaking time: 1–2 hours
Chilling time: 1 hour
Makes 4 individual tarts

INGREDIENTS

For the base:

- 70 g almonds
- 70 g desiccated coconut
- 60 g dates, pitted
- 1 tbsp coconut oil
- 1 tbsp lemon juice
- 1 tbsp vanilla extract
- zest of 1 lemon
- pinch of sea salt

For the filling:

- 60 g xylitol
- 200 g cashew nuts (soaked for 1–2 hours then drained and rinsed)
- pinch of sea salt
- 1 tsp baobab powder
- pinch of turmeric powder
- 1 tsp inositol powder
- juice and zest of 2 lemons
- juice of 2 limes

To garnish:

- a little lemon zest or coconut flakes

PER TART	
Calories	601 kcal
Protein	14.1 g
Total Fat	47 g
Saturates	16.8 g
Carbohydrates	35.9 g
Sugar	14.2 g

Line four individual tart tins with removable bases with cling film.

To make the base, process the almonds and coconut in a food processor until broken into a fine crumb. Add the remaining ingredients and process until the mixture comes together.

Divide the mixture between the tart tins and press down firmly. Place in the fridge and chill while making the filling.

For the filling, place the xylitol in a high speed blender or food processor and grind up until fine. Add the remaining ingredients and process until thick and smooth. Spoon the filling into the tarts and chill for 1 hour. Garnish with a little lemon zest and/or coconut flakes and serve.

CHAPTER TWELVE

Fertility-influencing Conditions

There are certain underlying conditions affecting a woman that can have an impact not just on her natural fertility, but also in some cases on the odds of IVF working, depending upon the severity of the condition affecting her. We don't often think of specific nutritional changes being able to target specific fertility conditions, but in fact there is a lot a woman can do to help minimise the effect of such conditions on her body and maximise her chances of fertility success.

POLYCYSTIC OVARY SYNDROME

Polycystic ovary syndrome (PCOS) is a condition that affects approximately 5–10 per cent of women in the western world, and I see it cause so much anguish for women in my clinic. (A greater number – around 20 per cent – may have a tendency towards polycystic ovaries, which is a different, usually less complicated condition that doesn't tend to affect fertility.) PCOS usually occurs because a woman's ovaries are unable to produce hormones at the right levels at the right times in her cycle. In particular luteinising hormone (LH) may remain high throughout a menstrual cycle and she may have raised testosterone levels. The result of these imbalances, and the presence of cysts, is that eggs don't fully mature within the ovarian follicles, and the follicle may fail to release them even if they do.

It's also worth thinking back a step further – what causes the hormone imbalance? There are all sorts of ways in which our lifestyle and other factors affect hormone balance, not least stress (see pages 42–5). Furthermore, blood sugar imbalances, and even insulin resistance (insulin is the hormone your body releases in response to sugar levels in your blood), can lead to high levels of testosterone, which can be damaging to eggs.

As a result, one of the best ways to use your diet to improve symptoms and effects of PCOS is to ensure it is blood sugar balancing. This means eating foods that sustain energy output in your system, rather than causing energy peaks and troughs. Opt for slow-releasing carbohydrate foods (those with a low GI; see page 66), as well as a diet relatively high in healthy proteins and low in saturated fats. Daily exercise is also important as this will help to keep your weight under control if this is a problem for you: 20 minutes of brisk walking (or equivalent) three times a week is all you need to aim for, especially if you aren't used to taking regular exercise.

As well as a daily multivitamin supplement, inositol and folic acid supplements have been shown in studies to help reduce the effects of PCOS (see pages 74–5 for specially formulated supplements). Taking a folic acid and inositol supplement at least one month before beginning your IVF treatment, but ideally for three months before, can help to regulate your insulin levels and balance out testosterone and progesterone in your system. Although inositol is available in your diet, it's such an important nutrient in the management of PCOS that supplementation is likely to be the best way to use this nutrient to improve your chances of conceiving. Our studies show that 4 g of myo-inositol powder every day can increase the number of eggs available for harvesting and improve subsequent fertilisation rates. (See the full range of Zita West products at www.zitawest.com.)

ENDOMETRIOSIS

Approximately 1 in 10 women of reproductive age in the UK suffer with some degree of endometriosis, a condition in which cells from the womb lining (the endometrium) migrate and attach to other parts of the body and begin developing there. The new patches of endometrial tissue respond to the monthly hormone cycle in exactly the same ways as the endometrium in the womb – bleeding and regrowing month to month. However, because the blood can't flow away (through the vagina, as with a period), it builds up and stagnates, causing pain and discomfort and interfering with fertility. Patches of endometrial tissue can form anywhere outside the womb, but commonly occur in the fallopian tubes, in the neck of the womb and around the ovaries.

It is thought that there are many factors involved in endometriosis, but hormone imbalance (perhaps an excess of oestrogen) is almost certainly a contributory factor, as well as possibly problems with immune function and inflammation in the body. See page 190 for advice on how to improve hormone balance using your diet and pages 173–7 for advice on how to reduce inflammation.

THYROID PROBLEMS

Your thyroid gland is the control centre of your body's metabolism – it produces hormones (triiodothyronine and thyroxine – known as T3 and T4 respectively) that regulate how your body converts and uses energy sources from your food, along with myriad other metabolic processes. However, the thyroid doesn't produce hormones without its own trigger. That trigger is thyroid stimulating hormone (TSH), which is produced in the pituitary gland in the brain.

Around 5 per cent of women with fertility problems are thought to have an under-functioning thyroid (known as hypothyroidism and leading to low levels of T4), which may result in heavy or long periods and anovulation (failure to ovulate). On the other hand, an overactive thyroid (known as hyperthyroidism) may result in scant periods or absence of them altogether, again affecting fertility. Different reference ranges of thyroid hormones indicate to doctors how well in balance the thyroid is prior to starting a round of IVF. If unbalanced, thyroxine may be used prior to starting an IVF cycle and also to see if thyroid antibodies are present as these may affect the success of IVF treatment.

The production of TSH, and therefore of T3 and T4, relies upon good levels of the nutrient iodine in your body (see page 72), as well as of the antioxidant vitamins A, C, E and nutrients iron, selenium and zinc, and tyrosine, B vitamins and essential fatty acids. You can find out more about the food sources of these nutrients on pages 67–73.

RECIPES FOR HORMONE HEALTH

Follicular Fluid Boost

One for the ladies, this drink is rich in vitamin E, an important antioxidant nutrient found in the fluid of the follicle housing your egg. In addition, inositol and protein powders provide nourishment to the follicular fluid. Cantaloupe melon and citrus fruits are particularly high in myo-inositol and by using kefir you can improve absorption by maintaining optimum digestive health.

Preparation time: 5 minutes
Serves 2

INGREDIENTS

- 170 g cantaloupe melon
- 2 peaches, stoned and chopped
- 1 chopped and frozen banana
- 30 g vanilla or plain protein powder
- 1 tbsp inositol powder
- pinch of ground cinnamon
- 1 tsp chia seeds
- 1 tsp omega blended oil
- 250 ml kefir or coconut kefir
- 100 ml orange juice

PER SERVING	
Calories	278 kcal
Protein	17.7 g
Total Fat	8.7 g
Saturates	3.2 g
Carbohydrates	31.7 g
Sugar	29.5 g

Place all the ingredients in a blender and process until smooth.

Baked Eggs in Avocado with Chilli

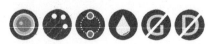

This is a simple nourishing breakfast option and is ideal for brunch, too. Eggs are rich in countless vitamins and minerals, including A, D, E, B2, B6, B9, iron, calcium, phosphorous, potassium and choline, which all contribute to a healthy reproductive system and hormonal balance. The choline and iodine in egg yolks are also crucial for making healthy thyroid hormones. The sprinkling of chilli seeds is a great way to boost your intake of beneficial omega fats. You could accompany this with wholegrain or rye toast if desired.

Preparation time: 15 minutes
Cooking time: 30 minutes
Serves 2

INGREDIENTS

- 2 tbsp mixed seeds (for example, pumpkin, sunflower and sesame)
- pinch of chilli flakes
- 1 tsp Worcestershire sauce
- drizzle of olive oil
- 1 avocado
- 2 eggs
- sea salt and black pepper

PER SERVING	
Calories	271 kcal
Protein	10.2 g
Total Fat	24 g
Saturates	4.8 g
Carbohydrates	3.5 g
Sugar	0.5 g

Preheat the oven to 180°C (gas mark 4).

Place the seeds in a small bowl with the chilli flakes, Worcestershire sauce, salt, pepper and olive oil. Toss together. Spread the seeds out on a baking tray and roast for 10–15 minutes stirring occasionally until golden. Set aside.

Cut the avocado in half, remove the stone and scoop a little extra of the flesh out, so you can fit the egg into it. Place the avocado halves in a small baking dish that fits them snugly so they won't move around.

Break the first egg into a bowl. Using a spoon, place the yolk in one half of the avocado, then carefully spoon over a little egg white (you may not manage to add all the white). Season with salt and pepper, then repeat with the other egg and the other half of the avocado.

Bake in the oven for 15 minutes, or until the white is opaque and the yolk is cooked lightly.

Serve the avocado on a plate with a scattering of the seeds on top.

Salmon Niçoise Salad with Herb, Caper and Walnut Dressing

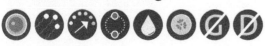

Summery and light tasting, this is a protein-packed salad full of beneficial omega-3 anti-inflammatory fats. Using walnut oil or an omega blend oil in the dressing is an easy way to further boost your intake of these healthy fats. This creamy dressing is equally delicious drizzled over any cooked fish or seafood. Rather than using traditional new potatoes I have opted for sweet potato here to provide plenty of carotenoids, which are valuable for improving sperm and egg health.

Preparation time: 15 minutes
Cooking time: 10 minutes
Serves 2

INGREDIENTS

For the salad:

- 1 small sweet potato, cut into large chunks
- 2 salmon fillets, about 120 g each, boneless, skin on
- 60 g French beans
- a handful of rocket leaves
- 30 g black olives, pitted
- 10 cherry tomatoes, halved
- 1 hard-boiled egg, cut into quarters

For the dressing:

- 2 tbsp walnut or omega blend oil
- 1 tbsp olive oil
- 2 tbsp capers
- juice of ½ lemon
- zest of 1 lemon
- 1 tsp Dijon mustard
- 2 tbsp chopped fresh herbs (for example, parsley and basil)
- sea salt and black pepper

PER SERVING	
Calories	574 kcal
Protein	29.8 g
Total Fat	40.6 g
Saturates	5.9 g
Carbohydrates	22 g
Sugar	7.4 g

Bring a large steamer to the boil, tip the sweet potato directly into the water, then lay the salmon fillets, skin-side down, in the steamer basket. Cover and cook for 6–8 minutes until the salmon is cooked through, then remove and set aside.

Add the French beans to the pan and blanch for 1–2 minutes then drain with the sweet potato.

Place the potato and beans in a large bowl and gently toss in the rocket, olives and tomatoes. Flake the salmon into large chunks, discarding the skin, and add to the salad along with the egg quarters.

Whisk all the ingredients for the dressing together. Season to taste and drizzle over the salad just before serving.

Chia Pots with Apricot Jam

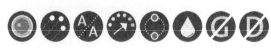

Apricots are an excellent fertility-boosting food as they are rich in beta-carotene and lycopene – important antioxidants known to help to improve sperm quality. Apricots also provide zinc, which is an important mineral for hormone production in both men and women. Chia seeds are packed with soluble fibre, protein and omega-3 fats to help stabilise blood sugar levels and support egg health. You can use kefir, whole milk or a milk alternative in this recipe. For a protein boost add a scoop of protein powder.

Preparation time: 10 minutes
Soaking time: overnight
Cooking time: 35 minutes
Serves 2

INGREDIENTS

For the apricot jam:
- 6 fresh apricots, stoned and chopped
- 2 tsp xylitol
- 1 scoop protein powder (optional)

For the chia pots:
- 4 tbsp chia seeds
- 300 ml kefir, whole milk or almond milk
- 250 ml Greek or coconut yoghurt

PER SERVING	
Calories	461 kcal
Protein	17.8 g
Total Fat	28 g
Saturates	12.9 g
Carbohydrates	38.5 g
Sugar	20.4 g

To make the apricot jam, place the ingredients in a pan with 60 ml of water and very gently simmer for 5 minutes or until the mixture is thick and syrupy. Place in a bowl in the fridge.

To make the chia pots, place the chia seeds in a jug with the milk. Stir well and leave to soak in the fridge overnight.

The next morning, place a little of the chia pudding in the bottom of two glasses. Top with a little of the apricot jam followed by a spoonful of yoghurt. Repeat the layers, finishing with the yoghurt, and serve.

Part 4

The Countdown Nutrition Plan

Any sustainable, meaningful change in the body takes time. This means that preparing your body for IVF treatment, and in the man's case preparing his sperm for fertilisation, is something that takes place over at least the three months running up to the first stages of the IVF process. No day is too soon or too late to begin – if you're already facing the start of your treatment, don't think that you're wasting your time adopting these measures now. Any time is a good time; the sooner, the better.

Throughout this section you'll find information about how to optimise your nutrition for IVF, balance your blood sugar and hormones, and reduce inflammation. This section also includes recipes to support your efforts as well as a 'Two week cleanse' that will prepare your body and nourish you before starting your cycle.

CHAPTER THIRTEEN

Clearing the System

In this chapter we'll look at a two-step process to get your gut health into optimal condition for treatment The first step is to start with a clean slate – giving your liver a chance to clear out the toxins and other residual nasties in your digestive system that could be impairing your gut health, without adding to the liver's load at the same time. This will immediately help to reduce any inflammation in your gut and give your immune system a boost. Second, we'll investigate the nutrients you should be increasing in your diet to ensure the best ongoing gut health possible.

Prior to IVF treatment we recommend you follow a cleansing programme for two weeks (see pages 148–51) to improve digestive function and liver function. Please note this is not a calorie restrictive detox diet – the aim of this process is to eliminate key known allergen foods, or foods that may promote inflammation in the body, and include foods known to support digestive health and liver detoxification processes.

Many organs are involved in the detoxification process, the main ones being the liver, the gastrointestinal mucosa, the skin, the lungs and the kidneys. These organs make use of various enzymes, transporters and elimination pathways to recognise and disable toxins. It is the liver which undertakes by far the greatest share of the work, through a process technically known as hepatic biotransformation, and we can support this through key nutrients in our diet. Crucial to detoxification is cell membrane health – since our cell membranes are composed of fatty acids, it is important to include plenty of healthy fats and phospholipids during the two-week programme.

To optimise liver function:

* Minimise toxins from food and drink – switch to organic foods where possible.
* Ensure a good supply of antioxidants to help disable the free radicals produced from our diet. At a low level they are a good thing but through a poor diet of processed foods, alcohol etc. the levels can increase, damaging all cells including sperm and egg cells. Antioxidants will help to neutralise them.
* Include plenty of leafy greens, berries and citrus fruits.

* Include protein at each meal. Sulphur amino acids are especially important in order for toxins to be excreted in the bile or urine. Good sources are lean organic or wild meat, game, poultry, fish, such as cod, salmon and trout, eggs and protein powders. Vegetarian sources of sulphur amino acids are eggs, nuts, seeds, beans and pulses. Aim for a palm-size portion (120 g) with each meal.

* Get a good supply of B vitamins for the detoxification process. This means aiming for at least 60–120 g of green leafy vegetables daily.

* Focus on digestive health which plays a key role in detoxification, so include fermented foods daily, such as probiotic yoghurts, kefir, nattō, tempeh and sauerkraut, and avoid foods known to aggravate the gut, such as gluten-containing foods (rye, wheat and barley).

* Ensure you open your bowels at least once a day – include foods that are rich in soluble fibre in your diet daily, such as beans, pulses, leafy greens, oats, wholegrain gluten-free grains, chia seeds, flaxseed, and apples and pears, which are rich in pectin fibre.

* Make use of therapies such as exercise and Epsom Salt baths to assist with detoxification. Exercise and movement are a very important part of the cleansing process and help to improve circulation, expel toxins and relax the body and mind by stimulating the release of endorphins.

* Before your daily shower, dry brush your skin from head to toe using small, quick circular movements. Brushing your skin for five minutes a day helps to increase circulation and break down fatty deposits within your body.

* Include a phospholipid supplement daily to support cell membrane health.

* Eat a wide range of brightly coloured fruits, vegetables, herbs and spices that are important for their phytochemicals known to help support detoxification pathways and reduce inflammation. These include cruciferous vegetables, pomegranate juice, berries, green tea, turmeric, ginger, onions, garlic, herbs such as coriander, dill, parsley, rosemary and mint, citrus zest and beetroot.

* Olive oil or other monounsaturated fats (MUFAs) should be your main source of fat. Also add polyunsaturated fats (PUFAs) from oily fish, nuts, seeds and cold pressed seed oils. MUFAs and PUFAs have been found to increase bile production, which is helpful for excreting the toxins produced during the detoxification process.

* Drink two litres of water or fluids daily – this can include green juices and smoothies, green tea, herbal teas, dandelion coffee, filtered water, coconut water, and nut or seed milks.

What to avoid during the two-week cleanse:

* Damaged fats – too much fried food and burnt food, especially well-cooked meat
* Gluten-containing foods, such as wheat, barley and rye
* Alcohol, smoking and recreational drugs
* Processed foods
* Coffee and regular tea – green tea is allowed as it is rich in antioxidants
* Larger cold water fish including shark, marlin, swordfish and tuna
* Exposure to toxins: use glass storage rather than plastic; glass, iron or ceramic cookware rather than non-stick, aluminium or stainless steel; and switch to glass or china in the microwave, rather than plastic

It is equally important to support digestive health. Some foods naturally contain enzymes that help to break down food in the gut. These include fresh pineapple (particularly the core), papaya and sprouted seeds. In addition, adding lemon or lime juice or vinegar to a meal can stimulate digestive secretions. This is why I recommend drinking a glass of warm water with the juice of half a lemon before meals.

Liver- and gallbladder-supporting foods

There are a number of foods that are known for their specific liver and gallbladder supporting properties. The following are included in the cleanse programme:

• Apples
• Asparagus
• Beetroot
• Artichokes
• Berries
• Bitter leafy greens, such as endive and chicory
• Brassicas, such as broccoli, Brussels sprouts, cabbage, cauliflower and watercress
• Celery
• Fennel
• Herbs, such as parsley and coriander
• Spices, such as garlic, ginger and turmeric

OPTIMISING THE SYSTEM

As well as following the advice for improving gut health on pages 105–6, include certain ingredients in your food that are known to have a positive effect on gut health:

* Cinnamon is known to help support digestion, by stimulating the digestive system encouraging it to function optimally.
* Fermented foods, such as kefir, sauerkraut, kimchi, kombucha, yoghurt, nattō, tempeh and raw pickled cucumbers, as well as garlic and beetroot all help to promote levels of good bacteria in the gastrointestinal tract.
* Bitter greens support digestive secretions. Try to include ingredients such as watercress, rocket and dandelion greens, as well as turmeric and fenugreek, in your dishes daily.
* A little lemon juice in warm water before meals will help to stimulate digestive secretions.

Always remember to eat mindfully – avoid eating on the go and chew your food properly (see page 106).

THE TWO-WEEK CLEANSE

Start each day with a glass of warm water with the juice of half a lemon added.

WEEK ONE

DAY ONE

Breakfast	Lunch	Dinner	Snacks (optional)
» Beet Burst Juice (page 220) » Cranberry and Walnut Granola Cluster (page 94) with a handful of berries and full-fat plain or coconut yoghurt	» Indian Spiced Cauliflower and Lentil Soup (page 179) » Turmeric Seeded Bread (page 121) spread with nut butter or houmous » Large mixed salad with lemon juice and olive oil	» Chicken Schnitzel with Beetroot and Apple Pickle (page 156) » Steamed broccoli, pak choi and carrots » Sweet potato wedges or baked sweet potato	» Lime and Avocado Smoothie (page 84) » Raspberry Mousse Pot (page 203)

DAY TWO

Breakfast	Lunch	Dinner	Snacks (optional)
» Acai Berry Seeded Smoothie (page 196) » Coconut Porridge with Berry and Cardamom Compote and Bee Pollen Sprinkle (page 85)	» Cleansing Broccoli Cream Soup with Hazelnut Sprinkle (page 197) » 2-egg omelette with raw sauerkraut and gluten-free oat cakes	» Chermoula-baked Salmon (page 91) » Wholegrain rice » Large mixed salad with lemon juice and olive oil	» Green Minted Cleanse (page 166) » Supergreen Flapjack Seed Bar (page 167)

DAY THREE

Breakfast	Lunch	Dinner	Snacks (optional)
» Vitamin C Kefir Strawberry Shake (page 109) » Supergreen Flapjack Seed Bar (page 167)	» Kale Hemp Pesto with Courgette and Carrot Noodles (page 128) » Slices of chicken breast or half a tin of cooked chickpeas	» Turkey San Choy Bau (page 221) » Large mixed salad with lemon juice and olive oil	» Chocolate Protein Bar (page 160) » Full-fat plain yoghurt with fresh berries

DAY FOUR

Breakfast	Lunch	Dinner	Snacks (optional)
» Deep Green Protein Shake (page 154) » Full-fat plain yoghurt with citrus fruits	» Jerk Chicken Salad with Avocado and Mango Salsa (page 216) » Turmeric Seeded Bread (page 121) spread with coconut butter or unsalted butter	» Grilled Sardines with Tapenade and French Beans (page 185) » Green salad » Cooked quinoa or buckwheat	» A handful of olives and vegetable sticks » Sun-dried Tomato Gluten-free Crackers (page 123) spread with nut butter

DAY FIVE

Breakfast	Lunch	Dinner	Snacks (optional)
» Follicular Fluid Boost (page 137) » Supergreen Flapjack Seed Bar (page 167)	» Roasted Squash Soup with Chipotle Cream (page 87) » Sun-dried Tomato Gluten-free Crackers (page 123) spread with nut butter » Mixed salad with half a tin of cooked beans or 120 g of grilled tofu	» Fish Tagine with Green Olives and Preserved Lemon (page 100) » Wholegrain rice » Green salad	» Raspberry Mousse Pot (page 203) » Vegetable sticks and houmous

DAY SIX

Breakfast	Lunch	Dinner	Snacks (optional)
» Coconut Porridge with Berry and Cardamom Compote and Bee Pollen Sprinkle (page 85)	» Roasted Root Vegetable, Tomato and Lentil Salad with Lemon Tahini Dressing (page 89) » Turmeric Seeded Bread (page 121) spread with coconut butter » Green side salad	» Roast chicken with steamed broccoli, asparagus and carrots » Baked sweet potato	» Speedy Smoked Mackerel Pâté (page 213) with oat cakes » Chopped apple or pear with full-fat plain or coconut yoghurt

DAY SEVEN

Breakfast	Lunch	Dinner	Snacks (optional)
» Green Minted Cleanse (page 166) » Frittata Traybake (page 199)	» Salmon Niçoise Salad with Herb, Caper and Walnut Dressing (page 140) » Oat cakes or gluten-free seeded crackers	» 2-egg omelette with Red Rice, Quinoa and Feta Salad with Pomegranate and Pistachios (page 218)	» Mixed berries with full-fat plain yoghurt » Follicular Fluid Boost (page 137)

WEEK TWO

DAY ONE

Breakfast	Lunch	Dinner	Snacks (optional)
» Chia Pots with Apricot Jam (page 142)	» Roasted Tomato, Tortilla and Chicken Soup (page 96) » Large mixed salad with lemon juice and olive oil	» Miso Glazed Cod with Sesame Seeds and Wilted Pak Choi (page 114) » Steamed broccoli » Green leafy side salad	» Turmeric Anti-inflammatory Blast (page 178) » Vegetable sticks with nut butter

DAY TWO

Breakfast	Lunch	Dinner	Snacks (optional)
» Deep Green Protein Shake (page 154)	» Salmon Niçoise Salad with Herb, Caper and Walnut Dressing (page 140)	» Turkey San Choy Bau (page 221) » Wholegrain rice	» Dreamy Salt and Vinegar Kale Crisps (page 169) » Chocolate Protein Bar (page 160)

DAY THREE

Breakfast	Lunch	Dinner	Snacks (optional)
» Follicular Fluid Boost (page 137)	» Baked Eggs in Avocado with Chilli (page 138) » Mixed salad with lemon juice and olive oil	» Baked Sea Bass with Salsa Verde (page 171) » Steamed broccoli, cauliflower and green beans » Baked sweet potato	» Supergreen Flapjack Seed Bar (page 167) » Berries and full-fat plain yoghurt

DAY FOUR

Breakfast	Lunch	Dinner	Snacks (optional)
» Vitamin C Kefir Strawberry Shake (page 109) » Supergreen Flapjack Seed Bar (page 167)	» Jamaican Jerk Veggie Burgers with Carrot and Celeriac Slaw (page 126) » Mixed salad with lemon juice and olive oil	» Grilled Sardines with Tapenade and French Beans (page 185) » Mixed salad with lemon juice and olive oil	» Raw sauerkraut and gluten-free seeded crackers » Turmeric Anti-inflammatory Blast (page 178)

DAY FIVE

Breakfast	Lunch	Dinner	Snacks (optional)
» Cranberry and Walnut Granola Cluster (page 94) with fresh fruit	» Malaysian Mee Goreng (page 124)	» Chicken Schnitzel with Beetroot and Apple Pickle (page 156) » Steamed vegetables	» Chocolate Protein Bar (page 160) » Dreamy Salt and Vinegar Kale Crisps (page 169)

DAY SIX

Breakfast	Lunch	Dinner	Snacks (optional)
» Chocolate Protein Bar (page 160)	» Kale Hemp Pesto with Courgette and Carrot Noodles (page 128) » 2-egg omelette	» Garlic Baked Chicken with Romesco Sauce (page 98) » Steamed vegetables » Mixed salad with lemon juice and olive oil	» Lime and Avocado Smoothie (page 84) » Raspberry Mousse Pot (page 203)

DAY SEVEN

Breakfast	Lunch	Dinner	Snacks (optional)
» Deep Green Protein Shake (page 154)	» Jerk Chicken Salad with Avocado and Mango Salsa (page 216) » Gluten-free seeded crackers	» Chermoula-baked Salmon (page 91) » Sweet potato wedges » Steamed vegetables	» Berries with a handful of nuts » Chilli Sweet Potato Chips with Avocado Ranch Dip (page 201)

CHAPTER FOURTEEN

Balancing Your Blood Sugar

The term 'blood sugar' relates to the amount of glucose in your bloodstream at any one time, which in turn affects your energy levels. For good health aim to keep your blood sugar balanced throughout the day – this will help to ensure stable energy levels and stable metabolic processes. A diet high in refined carbohydrates (such as white bread, rice and pasta, as well as refined sugars), sugary drinks and processed foods can lead to blood sugar imbalance (manifesting as peaks and troughs of energy throughout the day), which in turn has a negative impact on the health of your reproductive system.

Low blood sugar (which will make you feel lethargic) stimulates the body's release of stress hormones (adrenaline and cortisol). Continued release of stress hormones alters the way in which your body responds to progesterone, which is so important for the proper function of the menstrual cycle (see pages 8–10). High blood sugar (that sugar high burst of energy), when frequent and sustained, causes the body to release the hormone insulin, which aims to get sugar levels under control. The trouble is that if we have too much insulin in our system too frequently, the insulin receptors in the body (some of which are on the ovaries) begin to desensitise, creating a condition called insulin resistance. This is a major risk factor for PCOS (see page 134), and may even directly cause damage to a woman's eggs.

So, one way or another, keeping your blood sugar under control is essential for optimising your chances of pregnancy, whether through IVF or naturally. The best way to do this is to eat low-GI foods rich in protein and healthy fats, aiming for whole grains and starchy vegetables, such as sweet potato, carrots and beetroot, to help stabilise blood sugar levels. It's also important to eat regularly to avoid long periods of time without eating so you don't hit the energy slump that might send you reaching for unhealthy sugary foods. If you have followed the two-week cleanse, this will have helped with balancing your blood sugar.

WHAT ABOUT A SWEET TOOTH?

If you crave chocolate and sweets, I don't believe that your diet should be about complete denial. Rather than thinking you must cut out all sweet foods, try to think about how you satisfy your need for something sweet. Avoid the usual cakes and biscuits and try to include healthier options (such as Chocolate Protein Bars (page 160) or Cherry and Apple Crisp (page 118)).

* Have a couple of squares of dark chocolate (with at least 70 per cent cocoa solids) to satisfy chocolate cravings.
* Choose one of our protein smoothies – sweet and fruity but with healthy fats and protein to stabilise blood sugar levels (see page 154 for our Deep Green Protein Shake).
* Have a piece of fruit with some nuts to provide protein and stabilise blood sugar levels.
* For baking choose polyols (reduced-calorie carbohydrates) like xylitol, which is a low-calorie natural sweetener (derived from birch), or stevia (derived from the plant).

If you usually have sugar in your tea or coffee (bearing in mind you should minimise your intake of caffeine-containing drinks while you're trying for a baby anyway), don't be tempted to reach for artificial sweeteners, which are often made using some chemical nasties that can upset your body's systems. Try instead to adjust your palate, gradually reducing the amount of sugar you take until you're used to drinking coffee and tea without it.

Don't be fooled into thinking that syrups and honey are healthier – they are still forms of sugar. Overall, cut back on sweet foods where you can. Take a look at the recipes that follow for meals that contain just the right amounts of complex carbohydrate and slow-release energy foods to keep your blood sugar levels stable.

RECIPES FOR BLOOD SUGAR BALANCE

Deep Green Protein Shake

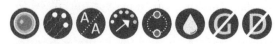

This is the perfect cleanse breakfast drink or healthy snack. By adding spirulina you provide valuable protein, essential fats and key nutrients for egg and sperm health, including B vitamins, manganese, selenium and zinc. Packed with antioxidants, this smoothie can help protect the body from free radical damage as you prepare your body for pregnancy.

Preparation time: 5 minutes
Serves 2

INGREDIENTS

- 2 Brazil nuts
- 1 nori sheet, torn
- 1 ripe banana
- 150 g frozen berries
- 2 handfuls of spinach leaves
- a handful of kale
- 250 ml almond or whole milk
- 1 tsp chia seeds
- 30 g vanilla or plain protein powder
- 1 tsp spirulina

PER SERVING	
Calories	176 kcal
Protein	15 g
Total Fat	3.5 g
Saturates	0.2 g
Carbohydrates	20.9 g
Sugar	13.7 g

Simply place all the ingredients in a blender and process until smooth and creamy.

Health benefits

Brazil nuts are a rich source of selenium, an antioxidant which is essential for sperm formation and testosterone production. Low levels of selenium are associated with poor motility of sperm. The addition of nori is a simple way to boost iodine intake, which is known for its role in healthy egg development.

Breakfast Burrito with Pesto

Breakfast burritos are a great way to provide plenty of protein and slow-releasing carbs with the added benefit of being easy to grab and go: simply wrap in baking parchment and pack in a container to take with you. Make sure you choose wholegrain or seeded wraps for additional fibre. Gluten-free wraps are also readily available.

Preparation time: 15 minutes
Cooking time: 4 minutes
Serves 2

INGREDIENTS

- 4 eggs
- 2 tbsp pesto
- 1 tbsp butter or coconut oil
- 1 tomato, diced
- 2 handfuls of baby spinach leaves
- 2 wholegrain, seeded or gluten-free wraps
- 30 g feta cheese, crumbled
- sea salt and black pepper

PER WRAP	
Calories	507 kcal
Protein	23.6 g
Total Fat	30.7 g
Saturates	10.6 g
Carbohydrates	33.5 g
Sugar	2.8 g

Beat the eggs with the pesto in a bowl and season. Heat the butter or coconut oil in a frying pan and pour in the eggs. Stir frequently until the eggs are scrambled to your liking, about 2–3 minutes. Remove from the pan.

Add the tomato and spinach to the pan and heat through to wilt the spinach – this should take about a minute.

Warm the wraps according to the packet instructions. Place one tortilla on a work surface and arrange half of the egg mixture in a line down the middle. Arrange half of the spinach and tomato mixture alongside the eggs. Sprinkle half of the feta cheese over the top.

Roll the wrap up to form a burrito and cut it in half horizontally. Repeat with the remaining wrap and serve.

Chicken Schnitzel with Beetroot and Apple Pickle

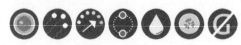

In this take on an Austrian classic, chicken breasts are tenderised then coated with a spicy nutty crumb to create a deliciously crispy fillet. These could be sliced and served cold with a salad for an easy prepare-ahead lunch or you could also try drizzling over a little barbecue sauce (page 214) for an extra spicy kick. The fruity Beetroot and Apple Pickle is packed with beneficial bacteria to support digestion and immune health.

Preparation time: 15 minutes
Cooking time: 6 minutes
Serves 2

INGREDIENTS

- 2 chicken breast fillets, about 120 g each, boneless and skinless
- 100 g ground almonds
- 30 g Parmesan
- ½ tsp smoked paprika
- ½ tsp garlic powder
- 1 egg, beaten
- a little plain flour or gluten-free flour, for dusting
- 1 tbsp coconut oil
- a little olive oil, for brushing (if oven cooking)
- sea salt and black pepper
- Beetroot and Apple Pickle (page 110), to serve

PER SERVING	
Calories	615 kcal
Protein	50 g
Total Fat	40.1 g
Saturates	8.9 g
Carbohydrates	13.6 g
Sugar	11.4 g

If you would prefer to cook the chicken fillets in the oven rather than pan-frying them, preheat the oven to 180°C (gas mark 4).

Place a layer of cling film on your work surface and place the chicken fillets on top. Cover the fillets with another piece of cling film and, using a rolling pin, bash the chicken until it is 2–3 mm thick.

Combine the ground almonds, Parmesan and spices in a shallow bowl and mix well. Season well with salt and pepper.

Place the beaten egg in a separate shallow bowl.

Dust the chicken fillets in a little flour. Dip the chicken in the egg and then coat thoroughly in the spice mixture.

Heat the coconut oil in a large frying pan and sizzle the chicken fillets for 2–3 minutes each side until golden and cooked through. Alternatively, brush the fillets with a little olive oil, place on a baking tray and cook in the oven for 15 minutes or until cooked through.

Serve with a generous helping of Beetroot and Apple Pickle.

Nutella Chocolate Protein Cookies

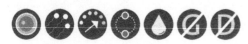

A perfect sweet treat to satisfy cravings and provide a wealth of healthy fats and protein to support healthy egg development. Hazelnuts are rich in protein, dietary fibre, iron, calcium and vitamin E. Vitamin E has been shown to enhance sperm binding to the egg and reduce sperm DNA damage.

Preparation time: 15 minutes
Cooking time: 18 minutes
Makes 12 cookies

INGREDIENTS

- 125 g hazelnuts
- 30 g coconut oil, melted
- 30 g protein powder
- 30 g cocoa powder
- 1 egg
- ½ tsp baking soda
- ½ tsp salt
- ½ tsp baking powder
- 1 tsp vanilla extract
- 2 tbsp xylitol
- 35 g sugar free dark chocolate chips

PER COOKIE	
Calories	137 kcal
Protein	4.5 g
Total Fat	11 g
Saturates	3.6 g
Carbohydrates	5.6 g
Sugar	2.5 g

Preheat the oven to 180°C (gas mark 4). Line a baking tray with baking parchment.

Place the hazelnuts in a food processor and grind until fine. Add the remaining ingredients, except the chocolate chips, and process briefly to form a thick batter.

Stir in the chocolate chips.

Take spoonfuls of the mixture and shape into round cookies. Place on the baking tray.

Bake in the oven for 15 minutes or until lightly golden and firm to the touch. Allow to cool on the tray for 5 minutes before removing to cool on a wire rack.

Chocolate Protein Bars

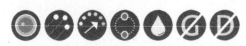

These no-bake bars can be thrown together in minutes and they make the perfect grab-and-go breakfast or snack. This is a high-protein bar packed with superfoods to nourish the body and support adrenal health. The combination of pecan nuts and almonds gives these bars plenty of healthy fats and protein as well as essential fertility-boosting nutrients, B vitamins, folic acid, zinc and vitamin E.

Preparation time: 15 minutes
Chilling time: 1 hour
Makes 8 bars

INGREDIENTS

- 120 g chocolate protein powder
- 30 g coconut flour
- 1 tsp cinnamon
- 1 tsp maca powder
- 1 tbsp inositol powder
- 1 tbsp raw cacao powder
- 1 tsp vanilla extract
- 3 tbsp honey
- 100 ml whole or almond milk
- 30 g coconut oil, melted
- 75g cashew or almond nut butter
- 50 g sugar-free dark chocolate chips

PER BAR	
Calories	134 kcal
Protein	13.2 g
Total Fat	2.8 g
Saturates	1.4 g
Carbohydrates	13.7 g
Sugar	7.3 g

Grease and line a 20-cm square baking tin with baking parchment.

Place all the dry ingredients, except the chocolate chips, in a food processor and combine. Add the remaining wet ingredients and process to form a stiff dough. Stir in the chocolate chips.

Press the mixture firmly into the baking tin using the back of a spoon.

Place in the freezer to firm up-then place in the fridge until required. Cut into bars and serve.

Cayenne Spiced Mixed Nuts

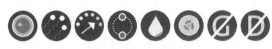

'Activating' nuts basically means that nuts are soaked and then dried to remove enzyme inhibitors which can make nuts difficult to digest. In this recipe the nuts are tossed in a spicy coating before toasting. These are an ideal snack to eat during the day and are a great way to cram in plenty of healthy fats and protein to energise the body.

Preparation time: 15 minutes
Soaking time: 4–6 hours or overnight
Cooking time: 17 minutes
Serves 6

INGREDIENTS

- 125 g mixed nuts (for example, cashew, Brazil nuts, hazelnuts, almonds, pecans)
- 1 tsp unsalted butter or coconut oil
- ¼ tsp cayenne pepper
- 1 tsp fresh rosemary, chopped
- 1 tsp coconut sugar
- 1 tsp sea salt

PER SERVING	
Calories	139 kcal
Protein	3.6 g
Total Fat	12.7 g
Saturates	2.9 g
Carbohydrates	2.6 g
Sugar	1.2 g

Place the mixed nuts in a jug or bowl and cover with filtered water. Soak for 4–6 hours or overnight.

Preheat the oven to 150°C (gas mark 3).

Drain and rinse the nuts and place on a roasting tray.

Heat the butter or coconut oil in a pan and add the cayenne pepper, rosemary, sugar and salt. Stir for 1–2 minutes until the sugar has dissolved. Pour the mixture over the nuts and toss to coat.

Place in the oven and bake for 15 minutes stirring occasionally until the nuts are lightly golden. Allow to cool then place in an airtight container until required.

CHAPTER FIFTEEN

Your Acid–Alkaline Balance

The human body constantly produces acids as a natural by-product of metabolism. However, for optimum health the body needs to maintain a slightly alkaline pH, which means it needs to buffer or neutralise excess acid in the system.

In terms of fertility, remember that sperm thrive in an alkaline environment – they are created in one and a woman's vaginal secretions are slightly alkaline to help ensure safe passage for the sperm within the female body. Recent research suggests that in general all cells (including the cells of an egg and then an embryo) prefer to grow in a slightly alkaline environment. Slight alkalinity is also better for your liver, encouraging it to function efficiently, ridding your body of toxins, and helping to maintain a good balance of healthy bacteria in your gut.

HOW TO EAT WITH ALKALINITY IN MIND

There are certain dietary principles that will help to keep your acid–alkaline balance in check. First, reducing the amount of caffeine, refined carbohydrates, processed foods, sweeteners or any foods you are allergic to in your diet will relieve the body of stress. Focusing more on plenty of plant-based proteins (for example, nuts, seeds, beans and pulses) and reducing your intake of red meat, as well as consuming plenty of vegetables, will help address the balance.

Learn to recognise foods that increase alkalinity, although it's not always straightforward to do so. For example, you might think that acidic foods, such as citrus fruits, are themselves acid-forming in the body, but in fact the opposite can be true: lemons, for example, have the effect of improving alkaline levels. As a general rule of thumb, though, vegetables, particularly leafy green vegetables, fermented foods, seeds, nuts and pseudo grains, like millet and quinoa, are good options.

Of course, it would be unrealistic to imagine that you're going to eat an alkaline-only diet and, besides, a balanced diet is always the healthiest option. As you embark upon your IVF treatment programme aim for 70 per cent alkalising foods in your diet and 30 per cent mildly acid-forming foods – that means good-quality protein is fine, but continue to avoid the dietary nasties of highly refined and processed foods.

ALKALISING SUPERFOODS

The following foods are well known for their detoxifying properties, which means that they support liver function and have an alkalising effect on the body. They all also contain wellness-promoting antioxidants, as well as other important nutrients for your fertility health. Include them in your cooking whenever you can – many of them will make wonderful additions to salads and 'green' juice blends.

* **Dandelion**
  Dandelion leaf and root provide an array of vitamins and minerals, as well as carotenoids and many other health-giving phytonutrients. Dandelion is also known for its supportive role in detoxification and maintaining a healthy liver, primarily due to a supportive influence on bile flow.
* **Watercress**
  In addition to its remarkable concentration of health-promoting vitamins, minerals, carotenoids and flavonoids, watercress is a potent source of sulphur compounds associated with healthy detoxification processes, such as glucosinolates.
* **Kale and other leafy greens**
  Research suggests that the major sulphur-rich antioxidants, such as sulforaphane and indole-3-carbinol, found in leafy greens may encourage the healthy elimination of various toxins that are known to be harmful to the liver.
* **Brassicas**
  Brassicas such as broccoli, cauliflower and cabbage ...
* **Parsley**
  In addition to its historical use as a tonic for kidneys and the urinary tract in general, parsley also provides an abundance of chlorophyll, which may contribute to a healthy digestive environment.
* **Beetroot**
  Beetroot provides various B vitamins and significant levels of vitamin C, the minerals potassium, iron, zinc, magnesium and copper, and the

important methyl donor betaine (which plays a role in maintaining healthy liver function).

* **Burdock root**
One of burdock's major prebiotic compounds, inulin, is associated with maintaining a healthy intestinal environment and supporting healthy immune function. Burdock has also been used for centuries in Traditional Chinese Medicine for maintaining healthy detoxification and blood purification.

* **Nettle**
In addition to its traditional use in maintaining urinary tract function and the elimination of toxins, nettle is also one of nature's most concentrated sources of vitamins and minerals.

* **Turmeric**
The curcuminoids in turmeric have been researched for their powerful antioxidant properties, which is especially significant considering the destructive effect of free radicals on liver health. More specifically, there is some evidence that turmeric may enhance the activity of two enzymes crucial to liver health, glutathione-S-transferase and UDP glucuronyl transferase.

* **Artichoke**
In addition to helping maintain healthy bile flow, studies suggest that artichoke leaf protects against free radical damage to the liver and may support proper liver cell regeneration. Artichoke leaf has also traditionally been associated with healthy fat digestion.

* **Coriander**
As well as its abundance of chlorophyll, vitamins and minerals, studies suggest coriander may help support the body's own natural ability to remove heavy metals.

* **Vanilla**
Vanilla not only provides flavour to food, it may also have antimicrobial properties and is rich in antioxidants that fight free radicals.

* **Cinnamon**
Cinnamon cleanses and detoxifies, protects against free radical damage and helps to regulate blood sugar levels.

* **Flaxseed**
Flaxseed provides the body with soluble fibre to aid excretion.

* **Probiotics**
These can be added to your diet to support digestion and the elimination of toxins.

* **Royal jelly and bee pollen**
  Traditionally thought to aid fertility, these natural bee products also help to nourish the body.
* **Supergreen powders**
  Superfoods such as wheatgrass, chlorella and spirulina ...
* **Green tea**
* **Ginger**
* **Garlic**

What makes the body acidic?

I want to stress that in terms of your fertility it's important not to get too hung up on how you add alkalinity to your diet. It's probably more important to think about how to reduce the acidic load. Foods high in refined sugar, excess protein (particularly too much red meat) and foods that contain trans (bad) fats that are high in cholesterol, such as those in margarines, all increase acidity in the body. Reducing these in your diet will become a natural side effect of eating more healthily for your fertility, without you needing to focus on increasing alkaline foods in your diet. The net result will be to generally improve your acid–alkaline balance. In addition, don't forget that stress itself is acid-forming, too!

RECIPES FOR ACID–ALKALINE BALANCE

Green Minted Cleanse

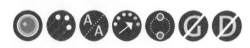

A refreshing. hydrating green juice packed with alkalising greens, this drink is ideal for the two-week cleanse (pages 148–51). Rich in B vitamins, including folic acid and inositol, it is ideal for supporting healthy eggs.

Preparation time: 5 minutes
Serves 2

INGREDIENTS

- 2 large handfuls of spinach leaves or kale
- 1 cucumber
- 1 lemon, peeled
- a large handful of fresh mint leaves
- 2 green apples
- 1 tsp omega blended oil or inositol powder
- ½ tsp superfood green powder

PER SERVING	
Calories	67 kcal
Protein	1.7 g
Total Fat	2.2 g
Saturates	0.2 g
Carbohydrates	9.5 g
Sugar	9.5 g

Place all the ingredients, except the oil and superfood powder, in a juicer.

Mix in the blended oil and superfood powder and divide between two glasses. If desired, top with ice.

Health benefits

Lemons are rich in vitamin C, a powerful antioxidant to protect against inflammation and damage to cells including sperm. Lemon juice is also incredibly alkalising and cleansing, supporting the liver, bile and digestion.

Supergreen Flapjack Seed Bars

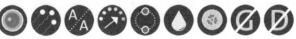

These light granola bars are packed with healthy fats, protein and essential minerals for supporting fertility. Ideal for a cleanse, they contain supergreen powder known for its cleansing and alkalising properties. They are perfect for a grab-and-go breakfast option or a healthy snack. The bars will keep in the fridge for one week or can be frozen for up to three months.

Preparation time: 15 minutes
Chilling time: 30 minutes
Makes 12 bars

INGREDIENTS

- 1 tsp vanilla extract
- 60 g wholegrain peanut butter or almond nut butter, no added sugar
- 60 g coconut oil
- 200 g soft pitted dates
- 125 g porridge or gluten-free oats
- 50 g walnuts
- 1 tsp superfood green powder (for example, blend, wheatgrass, spirulina or chlorella)
- 60 g pumpkin seeds
- 30 g sunflower seeds
- 2 tbsp ground flaxseed
- 1 tsp ground cinnamon
- 60 g dried cranberries or cherries

PER SERVING	
Calories	258 kcal
Protein	5.9 g
Total Fat	15.9 g
Saturates	5.7 g
Carbohydrates	22.6 g
Sugar	14.5 g

Line a 20-cm square baking tin with baking parchment.

Place the vanilla extract, nut butter, coconut oil and dates in a pan and heat gently to melt the oil. Place into a food processor and process until smooth.

Add the oats, walnuts, superfood powder and process to break up the nuts.

Add the remaining ingredients and pulse gently to combine. Do not overprocess as you want to retain some texture.

Press the mixture into the baking tin and place in the freezer for 30 minutes to firm up. Once chilled, cut in to bars.

Store in fridge until required.

Dreamy Salt and Vinegar Kale Crisps

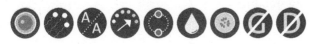

A wonderful healthy snack, these are ideal for the two-week cleanse (see pages 148–51). The crisps can be cooked in the oven or, if you have a dehydrator, you can dehydrate them overnight for a crispier texture. Using cashew nuts provides protein and zinc for the production of sex hormones including testosterone. Kale is an ideal cleansing leafy green vegetable, high in folic acid, iron (which promotes healthy red blood cells), calcium and manganese (a mineral recognised to help women get pregnant faster). You'll also find more than half of your daily vitamin A requirement in just one cup of kale. Baobab powder is a powerhouse of vitamin C – ideal for boosting immune health and antioxidant protection. Store the kale crisps in an airtight container. They will keep for 4–5 days at room temperature. If they soften you can crisp them up in the oven for a minute or two.

Preparation time: 10 minutes
Soaking time: 1 hour
Cooking time: 30–40 minutes oven cooking or 12–15 hours dehydrator
Makes 8 servings

INGREDIENTS

- 100 g cashew nuts (soaked for 1 hour then drained and rinsed)
- 1 tbsp baobab powder
- 1 tbsp inositol powder
- 1 tbsp nutritional yeast flakes
- 1 tsp sea salt or garlic salt
- 2 tbsp apple cider vinegar
- 200 g organic curly kale leaves, stalks removed, washed and chopped

PER SERVING	
Calories	97 kcal
Protein	3.9 g
Fat	6.5 g
Saturates	1.2 g
Carbohydrates	5.2 g
Sugar	2.8 g

If using an oven, preheat the oven to 120°C (gas mark ½) and line two baking trays with baking parchment. If using a dehydrator, line two teflex sheets.

Place the cashews, powders, yeast flakes, salt, vinegar and 100 ml of water in a blender and process until smooth.

Place the kale in a bowl.

Pour the sauce over the kale and massage into the kale with your hands ensuring it is evenly coated.

If oven cooking, spread the kale out on to the baking trays and bake for 30–40 minutes, stirring occasionally until the kale is crisp. If using a dehydrator, place the kale on the teflex sheets and place into the dehydrator. Dehydrate at 115°F for 12–15 hours or until crispy.

Baked Sea Bass with Salsa Verde

Salsa verde is a summery herb dressing and a perfect match for fish. Here watercress is added to the sauce for a peppery punch as well as providing valuable detoxifying nutrients, including B vitamins, zinc, potassium, vitamin E and vitamin C. This light, high-protein dish takes minutes to prepare and can be simply served with a mixed salad or steamed vegetables.

Preparation time: 10 minutes
Cooking time: 25 minutes
Serves 2

INGREDIENTS
- 1 whole sea bass, fins removed, cleaned and gutted
- 1 lemon, sliced
- sea salt and black pepper

For the salsa verde:
- 100 g watercress leaves
- 2 tbsp chopped fresh flat-leaf parsley
- 1 spring onion, roughly chopped
- 1 small garlic clove, roughly chopped
- zest of 1 lemon
- 1 tbsp capers, rinsed and drained
- 2 tbsp extra virgin olive oil

PER SERVING	
Calories	349 kcal
Protein	50.3 g
Total Fat	15.9 g
Saturates	2.5 g
Carbohydrates	1 g
Sugar	0.9 g

Preheat the oven to 180°C (gas mark 4). Line a baking tray with baking parchment.

Put the sea bass on the baking tray, stuff the lemon slices in the cavity and season with salt and pepper. Cover the fish loosely with foil. Bake for 10 minutes then remove the foil to uncover the fish and cook for a further 10–15 minutes until cooked through.

Meanwhile, to make the salsa verde, bring a small pan of salted water to the boil. Add the watercress leaves and cook for a minute. Drain and refresh the watercress in ice-cold water.

Transfer the watercress to a food processor, add the remaining ingredients and process to a purée. Season to taste with salt and pepper.

Place the sea bass on a large plate and peel back the skin. Pour over the salsa verde to serve.

CHAPTER SIXTEEN

Reducing Inflammation

Increasingly, all the roads to fertility point towards reducing inflammation in the body. It is not a problem for everybody, but for those who have specific inflammatory conditions or immune disorders (e.g.: lupus, crohn's disease, endometriosis) there is so much that diet and nutrition, including supplements, can do to help. This is one way you can really take control of your situation.

Inflammation is an immune system response – it signals that something is wrong with your body's systems and your body is working hard to put things right. When the immune system has done its work, the inflammation dies down and the body's natural balance is restored. In this respect inflammation is a good thing – a positive part of the healing process – and we should welcome it. However, modern lifestyles, including poor dietary choices, mean that for many people inflammation is less a specific response to a specific situation; instead, it is persistent and ongoing.

This is when the problems begin, because persistent, ongoing inflammation in the body leads to conditions that adversely affect fertility, including PCOS, endometriosis, pelvic inflammatory disease and autoimmune conditions (including allergies). It can also mean that conception occurs at the wrong time during a natural fertility cycle and this in turn can increase your risks of miscarriage.

DIETARY SOLUTIONS

There are certain foods that are inflammatory and others that help reduce inflammation in the body. Let's start with the good stuff. Try to increase the following in your diet, because these foods are anti-inflammatory:
* Oily fish – levels of omega-3 fatty acids in oily fish help to counteract the inflammatory effects of omega-6 fats that are found in most meat.
* Certain nuts, like macadamia nuts, which are high in omega-9 fats and seeds like flaxseed, chia and hemp.

* Fruit and vegetables – high antioxidant foods help stem the action of free radicals (see page 79), which cause inflammation. Orange and dark green vegetables are especially important for their beta-carotene levels.
* Olive oil, which in its raw state contains omega-9 healthy fats and a chemical called oleocanthal, both of which have anti-inflammatory actions on the body. However, once you heat olive oil it becomes pro-inflammatory, so opt for seed oils for cooking instead (see page 51).
* Spices such as turmeric, garlic and ginger help to prevent pro-inflammatory enzymes from acting on your body.
* Green tea is rich in anti-inflammatory.
* Pineapple compounds including catechins.
* Rosemary contains anti-inflammatory bromelain.
* Propolis (honey bee resin) is a source of caffeic acid phenethyl ester* (CAPE), which has been found to inhibit NF-kB, which promotes inflammation.
* Apples, onions, berries, brassicas and capers are a good source of quercetin, an important anti-inflammatory antioxidant.
* Fermented foods, such as kimchi, sauerkraut, kefir, kombucha and yoghurt, should be included regularly in your diet. The gut is an important site for the development and maintenance of immune health and modulating inflammation. Therefore maintaining a healthy digestion is important for addressing long-term inflammation.
* Collagen-rich bone broths
* Vitamin D-rich foods, such as oily fish, shellfish, egg yolk and mushrooms.
* Coconut oil contains a beneficial fatty acid called lauric acid, which is also found in human breast milk. Lauric acid converts in the body to a compound called monolaurin, which may help support the immune system. Other fatty acids include capric and caprylic acids, which have antimicrobial properties.
* Vitamin A-rich foods, such as organic liver and eggs.

In addition, try to eat more white fish, beans and pulses as your main protein sources, rather than poultry and red meat. Although turkey and chicken are fine in moderation, in general animal protein is considered more inflammatory for the body than fish and plant protein. You may wish to limit your

---

* contains a number of anti-inflammatory compounds including rosmarinic acid.

intake of red meat and dairy products, as they contain arachidonic acid, which the body can use to make inflammatory eicosanoids. You don't need to cut out meat altogether; just try to limit your intake to one or two times per week and focus on grass-fed and/or organic meats.

Unsurprisingly, the pro-inflammatory foods in our diet comprise refined carbohydrates and sugars, excess saturated fats, processed foods, junk foods and hydrogenised (or partially hydrogenised) fats. Avoid them as often as you can. Caffeine and alcohol are pro-inflammatory, too.

Finally, avoid stress. Although this isn't a dietary cause of inflammation, stress is almost certainly contributing to inflammation in your body. Support all the good work you're doing with your diet by adapting your lifestyle to reduce stress, too.

OPTIMISING YOUR IMMUNE SYSTEM

Before we get into how you can use your diet to bring your immune system into alignment, it can be helpful to understand how your immune system might affect conception.

The Zita West Fertility Clinic specialises in trying to understand the underlying reasons why IVF fails. Pregnancy is a unique phenomenon in the human body – a woman's body has to allow the foreign protein from a man's sperm to fertilise her egg. This requires a certain level of 'immune tolerance' in the woman's body. Some women, particularly those who have an overactive immune system, may need extra tests and treatment to create a situation in which their body develops the immune tolerance it needs to sustain a pregnancy.

Medical science provides us with a great many tests that enable us to deconstruct and decipher the goings-on in an individual's immune system. It also provides us with lots of medicalised means by which to regulate immunity for improved odds of success. However, I am a great believer that a combination of tailored diet, supplements and lifestyle can modulate the immune system naturally, restoring balance and reducing inflammation in the body.

Part of the work we do with IVF looks at blood clotting factors and the immune system which is like an army of white blood cells. We all have special immune cells, known as B cells, that manufacture antibodies to fight foreign invaders (disease). However, B cells don't work on their own. They have a bunch of hard-working antibody builders and on-the-ground fighters known as T helper cells to assist them. These cells themselves are made up of different types of worker, namely Th1 and Th2 cells, each with a specific role in the war against infection and inflammation. Th1 cells in effect 'kill' foreign invaders in a direct action. Th2 cells take a longer-term approach, manufacturing antibodies to inhibit infection and inflammation.

One of the tests we look at is a blood test for the ratio of Th1 and Th2 white blood cells. This gives us an indication of whether the immune system is overactive or not.

Lymphatic drainage

Your lymphatic system is an essential part of your immunity and lymphatic drainage helps to move toxins and 'excesses' (including excess hormones) through your body in order that they can find their way to your liver and be expelled. Before you begin your next round of IVF treatment, consider a lymphatic massage – a massage to your abdomen that can help improve this natural process and contribute to your body's ability to start again with a clean slate. (Lymphatic drainage massage is a useful technique before the first round of IVF, too, to help generally detoxify the body before beginning your protocols.)

DIET FOR IMMUNE BALANCE

As a rule of thumb the Mediterranean diet (see page 61), which is rich in fresh fruit and vegetables, provides the basic nutritional requirement for a properly functioning immune system. In particular, tomatoes contain a substance called lycopene, which has the effect of reducing inflammation. Note that levels of lycopene are actually better in cooked tomatoes than in tomatoes when they're raw – think pasta sauces! The Mediterranean diet is also high in healthy omega-3 fats and relatively low in meat protein, which also helps to keep inflammation in check.

Foods to avoid

All the dietary and lifestyle advice for reducing inflammation in your body, outlined earlier in this chapter, will also help to boost and balance your immune function. See pages 178–86 for anti-inflammation recipes.

High intake of the following foods may trigger an overactive immune response in the body. Try to minimise these in your diet while you're undergoing your IVF treatment, especially if you suffer from allergies or other autoimmune conditions, which are signs of immunity imbalance:

* Dairy products (for some)
* Gluten-containing foods (many grain-based foods)

* Processed foods
* Sugar
* Alcohol
* Caffeine
* Red meat
* Cured foods

Vitamin D and your immune system

Although research is in its infancy, scientists now believe that vitamin D has a very important role to play in the proper functioning of the immune system. Vitamin D affects the activation of T cells in response to infection. We manufacture vitamin D by the effects of sunlight on the skin, although it is also present in small amounts in some foods, including some fish (salmon, tuna and sardines are the best sources). Remember that you are not aiming to suppress your immune system in order to achieve pregnancy, but to modulate it to encourage its proper function – because when it's functioning properly it will naturally do what's needed to sustain a pregnancy.

RECIPES FOR REDUCING INFLAMMATION

Turmeric Anti-inflammatory Blast

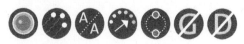

This is the perfect anti-inflammatory shake. Try including the core of the pineapple which contains the most bromelain, a digestive enzyme also known for its anti-inflammatory properties. If you can get hold of water kefir you can use this instead of coconut water to provide beneficial bacteria.

Preparation time: 5 minutes
Serves 2

INGREDIENTS

- 300 ml coconut water or water kefir
- 150 g pineapple, fresh or frozen, cut into chunks
- 100 g mango, cut into chunks
- 1 tsp coconut oil
- 1 tbsp inositol powder
- ½ tsp turmeric powder
- ¼ tsp ground ginger
- pinch of ground cinnamon
- pinch of black pepper
- 1 tsp bee pollen or Manuka honey
- 1 tsp probiotic powder (optional)

PER SERVING	
Calories	114 kcal
Protein	1.7 g
Total Fat	2.1 g
Saturates	1.4 g
Carbohydrates	22.1 g
Sugar	12.8 g

Place all the ingredients together in a blender and process until smooth and creamy.

Health benefits

Curcumin, the active component of turmeric, has been widely studied for its range of health benefits, notably its anti-inflammatory properties. The addition of fat and a pinch of black pepper to the smoothie aids the absorption of turmeric.

Indian Spiced Cauliflower and Lentil Soup

Soups are an easy way to cram in a lot of anti-inflammatory ingredients. This Indian-inspired cauliflower soup contains turmeric, garlic, onion and ginger – all known for their potent anti-inflammatory properties. Cauliflower is a wonderful addition in any detoxification plan too. Cauliflowers are part of the cruciferous family of vegetables known for being rich in compounds called glucosinolates which help support various detoxification pathways involved in eliminating toxins from the body. For a creamier texture you can blend the soup before serving.

Preparation time: 15 minutes
Cooking time: 45 minutes
Serves 2

INGREDIENTS

- 1 tbsp coconut oil
- 1 tsp cumin seeds
- 1 garlic clove, crushed
- pinch of sea salt
- ½ onion, finely chopped
- 1 celery stalk, finely chopped
- ½ tsp fresh ginger, grated
- ½ tsp turmeric powder
- ½ tsp curry powder
- 800 ml vegetable or chicken stock
- 60 g red lentils
- ½ head of cauliflower, broken into small florets
- 1 tbsp lemon juice
- 2 tbsp natural yoghurt, to garnish
- 1 tbsp fresh coriander leaves, chopped, to garnish

PER SERVING	
Calories	214 kcal
Protein	13 g
Total Fat	8.9 g
Saturates	5.9 g
Carbohydrates	21.2 g
Sugar	5.1 g

Heat the oil in a large saucepan over a medium heat. Add the cumin, garlic, salt, onion and celery and cook for about 3–5 minutes until softened.

Stir in the ginger, turmeric and curry powder and cook for about 30 seconds, until fragrant.

Stir in the stock and lentils. Cover and simmer until the lentils are tender – this should take about 20 minutes.

Once the lentils are soft, take the soup off the heat and, using a potato masher, break up the lentils. Return the pan to the heat, stir in the cauliflower and simmer for about 10 minutes or until the cauliflower is tender.

Divide the soup into two bowls, drizzle some lemon juice on top and garnish with the yoghurt and coriander leaves.

Steak Salad with Chimichurri Dressing

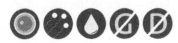

Chimichurri is a delicious spicy herb sauce ideal for serving with meats. It is packed with cleansing, antioxidant and anti-inflammatory ingredients making it a flavoursome, healthy dressing. For maximum flavour marinate the steak in a little of the sauce overnight. This is a fabulous energising, protein-packed dish ideal for a pick-me-up and for supporting flagging energy levels.

Preparation time: 15 minutes
Marinating time: 2 hours or overnight
Cooking time: 10 minutes
Serves 2

INGREDIENTS

For the chimichurri dressing:

- 1 garlic clove, crushed
- ½ red chilli, deseeded and chopped
- a large handful of fresh flat-leaf parsley leaves
- a handful of fresh coriander leaves
- pinch of ground cumin
- 30 ml apple cider vinegar
- 75 ml olive oil
- sea salt and black pepper

For the steak salad:

- 2 x 150 g lean beef fillet steaks
- 150 g bag of mixed salad leaves
- 4 radishes, sliced thinly
- ½ cucumber, cut in half lengthways and sliced
- 30 g chopped toasted cashew nuts

PER SERVING	
Calories	664 kcal
Protein	41.2 g
Total Fat	52.6 g
Saturates	10 g
Carbohydrates	5.3 g
Sugar	3.1 g

To make the dressing, place all the ingredients, except the salt and pepper, in a blender and process to form a chunky sauce. Season to taste.

Place the beef steaks in a shallow dish. Spoon a third of the dressing over the beef. Cover the dish tightly with cling film and marinate in the fridge for 2 hours or overnight, if possible.

Remove the beef from the fridge, discard the marinade and allow the steaks to reach room temperature.

Heat a griddle pan until hot. Season the steaks, then pan fry for 4–5 minutes on each side. Remove from the pan and allow to rest for 5 minutes. Slice thinly.

Pour the steak juices from the cooking pan into the remaining dressing.

Divide the salad leaves between two plates and top with the radishes and cucumber. Place the beef slices on top and scatter with cashew nuts. Drizzle over the dressing to serve.

Beef Massaman Curry with Cauliflower Rice

A flavoursome curry which is slow cooked and makes use of cheaper cuts of meat, this fork-tender dish is also packed with anti-inflammatory spices. The addition of coconut oil and milk provides plenty of lauric and caprylic acid to support a healthy immune response. Using cauliflower instead of refined white rice not only keeps this dish high in protein and lower in carbohydrates, but is an easy way to cram in more cruciferous vegetables in your diet, which are important for detoxification.

Preparation time: 20 minutes
Cooking time: 1 hour 7 minutes
Serves 2

INGREDIENTS

- 30 g unsalted cashew nuts
- 1 tsp coconut oil
- ½ tsp turmeric powder
- 2 tbsp massaman curry paste
- 250 g stewing beef steak, cut into large chunks
- 1 medium sweet potato, cut into chunks
- 4 shitake mushrooms, cut into quarters
- ½ red pepper, cut into chunks
- ½ onion, cut into thin wedges
- 2 kaffir lime leaves
- 1 tsp tamarind paste
- 2 tsp coconut sugar
- 1 tsp fish sauce
- 1 tsp tamari soya sauce
- 250 ml coconut milk
- 2 handfuls of baby spinach leaves
- ½ red chilli, deseeded and diced

For the cauliflower rice:

- ½ head of cauliflower, chopped
- 1 tbsp coconut oil
- 1 tbsp chopped fresh coriander leaves
- sea salt and black pepper

PER SERVING	
Calories	517 kcal
Protein	38.5 g
Total Fat	22.9 g
Saturates	9 g
Carbohydrates	39.3 g
Sugar	20.8 g

Place the cashew nuts in a frying pan and toast over a low heat until lightly golden. Set aside.

Heat the coconut oil in a large saucepan. Add the turmeric powder, curry paste and beef. Stir well and sauté for 1–2 minutes. Add the sweet potato, mushrooms, pepper, onion, kaffir lime leaves, tamarind paste, sugar, fish sauce and soya sauce. Pour over the coconut milk, stir well and bring to a simmer. Cover and cook gently for 1 hour until the beef is tender.

Turn off the heat and toss in the spinach and red chilli.

To make the cauliflower 'rice', place the cauliflower in a food processor and pulse into tiny fine rice-like pieces. Place a frying pan over a medium heat and add the coconut oil. Add the cauliflower and cook for 3–5 minutes until soft. Stir occasionally during cooking. Season and top with the coriander leaves.

Spoon the rice into bowls and top with the beef curry. Scatter over the cashew nuts to serve.

Grilled Sardines with Tapenade and French Beans

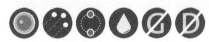

Sardines are an excellent source of omega-3 anti-inflammatory fats and protein, and are delicious served with this garlicky tomato tapenade. You can prepare the tapenade several days in advance. It is also wonderful as a healthy spread over crackers or wholegrain toast.

Preparation time: 15 minutes
Cooking time: 10 minutes
Serves 2

INGREDIENTS

For the tapenade:

- 8 cherry tomatoes
- 2 garlic cloves
- 1 tbsp olive oil
- 100 g pitted black olives
- 2 tinned anchovies, drained
- 2 tbsp capers, rinsed and drained
- 1 tbsp lemon juice
- 1 tbsp basil leaves, chopped
- pinch of black pepper

For the grilled sardines:

- 4 sardines, butterflied
- 100 g green beans, trimmed
- 1 courgette, sliced thickly diagonally
- ½ x 400 g tin cannellini beans, drained and rinsed

PER SERVING	
Calories	509 kcal
Protein	48.8 g
Total Fat	29.7 g
Saturates	7.2 g
Carbohydrates	11.6 g
Sugars	4 g

Preheat the grill to medium.

To make the tapenade, place the tomatoes on a baking tray with the garlic cloves. Drizzle over the olive oil. Place under the grill for 5 minutes until softened.

Add the tomatoes and garlic to a food processor with the olives, anchovies and capers. Gently pulse to combine but do not let the ingredients lose their texture entirely. Finish with the lemon juice, basil leaves and pepper.

Spread a little of the tapenade over the top of each of the sardines. Place on a baking tray and grill for 3–5 minutes or until golden and cooked through.

Meanwhile blanch the green beans and courgette in boiling water for 3 minutes then drain. Place back in the pan with the cannellini beans and the remaining tapenade and warm through.

Spoon the vegetables on to plates and top with the sardines to serve.

Part 5

Diet and Your IVF Cycle

Now that we've looked at how you can generally improve the quality of your diet in order to optimise your egg and sperm health, as well as how to best prepare the woman's body for receiving and accepting a fertilised embryo, it's time to move on to the specifics of the IVF process and how, week-to-week, phase-to-phase, you can use nutrition to further improve your chances of success.

There are no certainties with IVF, but it can be so empowering to know that you're doing all you can that's within your own sphere of control. This is where your diet and lifestyle come in. Throughout this section you'll find a detailed description of each stage of the IVF process, your body's needs at that particular time in terms of your nutrition and lifestyle, and recipes to help you keep on track and stay in control.

CHAPTER SEVENTEEN

Starting an IVF Cycle

Now you've balanced your hormones, blood sugar, sorted your gut health and inflammation in the run up to IVF and it's time to focus on each step of the process and how you can optimise it.

The women we see in the clinic are at all sorts of stages on their IVF journey when they arrive. Some have been through IVF before and are having to pick themselves up to begin again, while others are embarking on the journey for the first time, unsure of what the future holds. Either way, it's a stressful and uncertain process that can often feel out of your control. You do, however, have control over what you eat, what supplements you take, ensuring you get good amounts of rest and how you manage your stress levels.

THE START OF THE CYCLE

The majority of fertility clinics in the UK focus on the medical side of the IVF process. At the Zita West Fertility Clinic we prefer to take a more integrated approach, believing that while the medical aspects of treatment are of course imperative, it is equally important to think about nutrition and diet and the ways in which a couple can help themselves to optimise their chances of IVF success.

It's so important to bear in mind that it's not just that the woman needs to produce some eggs, but that those eggs need to mature fully and healthily; and that the man needs to produce sperm that have good quantity, motility and morphology. When I ask my clients who have gone on to have a successful pregnancy what they think made a difference, they so often list three things: I was less stressed; I rested more and looked after myself; and I changed my diet and improved my nutrition. This is what I want for every couple that picks up this book.

YOUR IVF CYCLE

The specific protocols for your IVF cycle will depend upon your particular clinic. However, all fertility clinics follow the same broad process for full IVF treatment:

* stimulation of your ovaries
* egg collection

* embryo transfer
  * the two-week wait (before you can take a pregnancy test)

We cover each of these phases in the treatment cycle in detail on pages 192–234.

GATHERING INFORMATION AND UNDERSTANDING THE TIMELINE

Without a doubt IVF is paper-driven. You will have huge amounts of information to take in – dates and times for appointments, and injections and scans to keep track of.

There are five key things I recommend you need to have in order before you start:

1) If you work, manage your working diary so that you can prioritise the time you'll need for your IVF treatment. The first two weeks of the schedule are the most intensive, with the most scans, appointments and procedures for egg collection and transfer.
2) Manage your expectations of how rigid your timeline will be: dates and times of appointments or injections and the day-to-day changes in your cycle can mean that sometimes things don't happen when you expect them. Aim to think and behave flexibly.
3) Learn some quick stress management strategies that you can use while you're waiting to be seen for your appointments – such as breathing in for the count of three and out for the count of five – because clinic appointments rarely run to time.
4) Organise yourself – set yourself little reminders on your watch or smartphone and keep a calendar. Remember that some of the injections you'll need to give yourself will have to be precisely timed – don't rely on your memory no matter how good you think it is. Be safe and write everything down and set alarms for precision timing.
5) Read all the information you're given – all of it, down to the last detail. Highlight passages that seem most important to you and ask questions about anything you don't understand. So many couples I see don't read everything, but being informed will make you feel more in control and less anxious about what's happening.
6) To get to the end of an IVF cycle and a transfer is great but there are lots of hurdles along the way. These include cysts which may stop you from starting a cycle, failure to down regulate, a poor response to treatment so your cycle is cancelled and poor fertilisation.

USING YOUR DIET

As you prepare for your IVF treatment to begin, do the two-week cleanse outlined on pages 148–51, which will improve your gut health and balance your blood sugar levels (see pages 105 and 152 respectively). Eat plenty of lean protein for egg and sperm building and focus on good fats (foods that are high in omega-3).

Focus on nutrition before IVF

- The most important step in downregulation is to manage stress and focus on foods to support hormone balance and lowering inflammation. Keep stress levels down and avoid processed foods, sugars, refined carbohydrates, alcohol and caffeine. Consider hypnosis and acupuncture to help get your stress levels down (see pages 46 and 47 respectively).
- Improve detoxification and your hormone balance: include soluble fibre – oats, flaxseed and chia seeds, leafy greens, garlic, onion and turmeric – in your diet.
- Support adrenal health: maca powder is a useful adrenal adaptogen herb and foods rich in magnesium are also important, for example halibut, leafy greens and pumpkin seeds.
- Keep inflammation in check (see pages 173–7).
- Keep your blood sugar levels balanced by eating regularly and including slow-releasing carbohydrates – starchy vegetables and whole grains like quinoa, millet, buckwheat and wholegrain rice – in your diet.
- Try adding bone broth to meals, warming soups and stews to nourish and keep stress levels in balance.

USING SUPPLEMENTS

This is an important time for preparing your body for conception and pregnancy. Take a multivitamin and -mineral, an omega-3 supplement and a vitamin D supplement. If your clinic considers you in the older category of women going through IVF, also take supplements of antioxidants, inositol and co-enzyme Q10. You will also benefit from an inositol supplement if you suffer from PCOS (see page 134).

Exercise and IVF success

For women, the kind of exercise you do and the amount you do can have a significant impact on the likelihood of IVF success. There can be no question that regular exercise, safely practised, is generally good for your health. Recent studies into the links between IVF success or failure rates and a woman's exercise levels suggest, however, that in order to optimise the chances of success, low-impact, moderate exercise for short periods of time is best. In particular, try to avoid running or impact sports and opt instead for walking, swimming or gentle yoga two or three times a week, for between 20 minutes and an hour at each session. It's important to maintain a healthy circulation and a healthy weight – being either overweight or underweight will in themselves reduce your chances of IVF success (see page 53).

In the lead up to an IVF cycle, we recommend no exercise for women other than walking while you're downregulating. Exercise during this time can be very depleting. Similarly, when you're going through the stimulation phase of treatment, your ovaries are enlarged so again it is not a good idea to exercise. Do keep moving though – walking will help maintain blood flow, nutrient flow and oxygen flow to your ovaries during stimulation. However, avoid impact exercise and yoga or Pilates which can cause torsion of the ovaries. Finally, we recommend no exercise after the transfer until the pregnancy is established, when you should exercise only under guidance from your medical team.

DOWNREGULATION

Not all women need to go through a downregulation phase but, if your IVF protocol includes it, this is when your natural menstrual cycle comes under medical control. Medications suppress the ovaries so that there is no activity in them from around Day 21 of your cycle. You'll have blood tests to measure your hormone levels as well as scans to see whether or not there is any activity in your ovaries so that doctors can tell whether or not you've downregulated. Many women feel tired during this phase and can be emotionally fragile, so don't push yourself and rest well. If you don't downregulate, which can happen, you may need to take medication in order to start your period so that your IVF cycle can begin.

Extra medication

As well as the routine IVF medications, your own medical situation may mean that you need to take additional drugs to bring other, underlying conditions under control and maximise your chances of success. Your clinic will let you know if this applies to you.

OVARIAN STIMULATION

If you are undergoing a downregulation protocol, once an ultrasound scan has confirmed that the first phases of treatment have been successful and the activity of your ovaries has been suppressed, your clinicians will confirm that you're now ready to move on to the stimulation phase of your IVF treatment cycle.

This is the most intensive part of the process when it comes to clinic appointments, scans and blood tests. You will need to begin by injecting a synthetic version of gonadotrophins (in a natural menstrual cycle, gonadotrophins would begin the maturation of the eggs) every day. Your clinic will show you how to do this, give you precise timings for when you should inject and will tell you how much you should inject. (The amounts may increase or decrease over the course of this phase, depending upon what your scans reveal about how many follicles have been stimulated.) Rest assured that the needle is tiny: once you've done it for yourself once, you'll be fine. This phase generally lasts between 10 and 12 days.

The scans you receive during this time will not only check follicular development, but also the thickness of your lining as it builds over the days. Your clinicians will want to know that it is on its way to reaching the appropriate thickness for implantation, should your eggs fertilise successfully.

> Try to rest as much as possible during this time. Don't over-exercise as the energy your body is using for the development of your follicles will make you tired. This might be a good time to try acupuncture to help manage your stress or give you energy.

Some women who have PCOS worry about overstimulation (a condition called ovarian hyperstimulation syndrome (OHSS); see page 27), but try not to worry. Your clinic should monitor you carefully which makes this unlikely. Furthermore, an early AMH test (see page 13) will help doctors decide before your treatment begins whether or not you're likely to develop OHSS and to medicate you appropriately if you are at risk.

USING YOUR DIET

You will have been nourishing your body in the lead up to IVF, so during this phase it's about making sure you have sufficient protein to build healthy eggs – remember IVF needs a lot of eggs! Choose lean, organic sources as often as you can. Energy-rich foods (such as iron-rich green leafy vegetables) are also good during this time. Mitochondria (see page 77) are developing inside your growing eggs and are essential for the health of your eggs and any potential baby. Iron is also good for helping the thickening of your womb lining. Healthy fats will help to promote good cell membranes within the eggs, and antioxidant foods will keep you fighting fit.

Follicular fluid

The follicular fluid that surrounds and nourishes the eggs is rich in beta-carotene, vitamins D and E, so increase foods containing these nutrients to help nourish the fluid and so nourish your eggs.

Good foods for stimulation

- Phospholipid-rich foods – soya, egg yolk, milk, lecithin granules, sunflower seeds
- Healthy fats – coconut oil, olive oil, avocado, nuts, seeds, nut butters, oily fish, omega blended oils for salad dressing, grass-fed or organic butter
- Vitamin D-rich foods – oily fish, shellfish, egg yolk, mushrooms
- Vitamin E-rich foods – almonds, sunflower seeds, leafy greens, avocado, fish, olive oil, butternut squash
- Beta-carotene foods – brightly coloured yellow and orange foods, leafy greens (for example kale and spinach)
- Lean proteins – fish, poultry, eggs, beans and pulses

USING SUPPLEMENTS
Try protein shakes at this time to promote blood flow and hence delivery of oxygen/nutrients.

CHAPTER EIGHTEEN

Egg Collection

After frequent monitoring and blood tests, your doctors will decide that your eggs have reached the point at which your follicles are ready to release them (see pages 8–9).

At this point you'll be given a 'trigger injection' of a drug that acts on the body in the same way as luteinising hormone (LH). Different clinics use different types of trigger injection. The timing of the injection is crucial – you will need to be in the clinic to have your eggs collected usually 34–38 hours later. Schedule all this in your diary and set your alarm (every alarm you have, if need be!) to remind you to take the injection at the right time. It's so easy during this very anxious part of the process to panic and forget. And if your precise time is during the night, there's every chance you may sleep through it – even if you think you won't.

Most clinics will advise you not to eat or drink anything after midnight the night before your eggs are due for collection: the collection procedure occurs under anaesthetic and having an empty stomach reduces the normal risks associated with general anaesthesia.

Unless you're using donor sperm, your partner will need to be with you at your collection appointment, so that he can provide a semen sample while your procedure is taking place. After that, he'll be able to stay with you to support you and to take you home afterwards. It's also important to manage your expectations about the number of eggs that your clinicians might collect. Not every follicle contains an egg – only once the doctors aspirate your follicles to collect the eggs can they tell for certain that eggs are inside. However, don't despair if you have only one or two eggs available for collection. Remember, it's about the quality of the eggs that the clinics collect and how well they have matured, not about the quantity. Your embryologist will grade your eggs and select those that are the most mature for the fertilisation stage of the process. Throughout the process, including the grading, your clinic will be in contact constantly to keep you updated and offer reassurance.

Usually there is very little pain once your anaesthetic has worn off and most women can manage any pain they do have (a bit like period cramping) with paracetamol. The more eggs that have been retrieved the more likely you are to have some pain. Finally, it's worth saying (by way of reassurance rather than alarm) that egg collection is an invasive procedure. You will feel tired and depleted after it has occurred. Your body will also need to heal before your embryos can be transferred and this should also inform how you approach your nutrition at this time.

USING YOUR DIET

Make sure you eat plenty of foods rich in vitamins C and E, which are essential for the body's healing mechanisms and will offer important antioxidant protection, post-operatively. Vitamin D-rich foods will help to support your immune system and foods rich in omega-3 fats will help to reduce any inflammation associated with having a surgical procedure. If you feel like treating yourself, eat lots of nourishing, comforting foods – tryptophan-rich foods that are good for feel-good hormones (see page 49) are a good choice. You should also aim to balance your blood sugar to keep stress levels down.

Good foods for egg collection

- Vitamin C-rich foods – red pepper, citrus fruits, berries, leafy green vegetables
- Magnesium-rich foods to modulate stress – spinach and leafy greens, beans and pulses, dark chocolate and raw cacao powder
- Zinc-rich foods – pumpkin seeds, fish, shellfish
- Omega-3-rich foods – oily fish, walnuts, flaxseed, chia, hemp seeds
- Vitamin E-rich foods – almonds, sunflower seeds, leafy greens, avocado, fish, olive oil, butternut squash
- Vitamin D-rich foods: oily fish, shellfish, egg yolk, mushrooms

---

USING SUPPLEMENTS

Supplements are an important part of any IVF programme alongside the correct diet. The roles of the nutrients zinc, selenium, iodine, vitamin D and omega-3 are well documented and there is an increasing body of evidence exploring the roles of other nutrients in relation to specific aspects of fertility including egg quality and sperm quality. We use supplements, general multivitamins and omega-3. In preparation for IVF we check vitamin D levels and supplement accordingly. Inositol is also used for certain women going through IVF and in preparation. Additional supplements will be used depending on the individual circumstance and any underlying conditions they might have.

To read more about our range go to www.zitawest.com

RECIPES FOR EGG COLLECTION

Acai Berry Seeded Smoothie

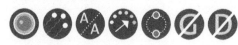

Antioxidant-packed and rich in anti-inflammatory fats to support cell health and follicle health, this delicious creamy shake will also boost your intake of beneficial bacteria.

Preparation time: 5 minutes
Serves 2

INGREDIENTS

- 300 g fresh or frozen berries
  (for example, strawberries, raspberries,
  blackberries, blueberries)
- 1 small banana, chopped
- 200 ml plain or coconut yoghurt or kefir
- 100 ml pomegranate juice
- a handful of spinach leaves
- 1 tsp goji berry or superberry powder
- 1 tsp acai berry powder
- 1 tsp probiotic powder
- 1 tbsp mixed seeds
- 30 g protein powder (optional)

PER SERVING	
Calories	354 kcal
Protein	21.8 g
Total Fat	16 g
Saturates	7.4 g
Carbohydrates	30.5 g
Sugar	27 g

Place the ingredients in a blender and process until smooth and creamy.

Health benefits

Pomegranates have long been a symbol of fertility. They are rich in many fertility-supporting nutrients, including vitamin C, vitamin K, folic acid and antioxidants. They have anti-inflammatory properties as well as helping boost blood flow to sexual organs.

Cleansing Broccoli Cream Soup with Hazelnut Sprinkle

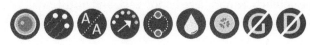

Avocados are rich in potassium, creating an alkaline environment, and broccoli contains fibre and glucosinolates, shown to support detoxification pathways and the elimination of toxins. Topped with a crunchy hazelnut sprinkle this is a light, yet creamy nourishing soup that is ideal for supporting a healthy detox.

Preparation time: 15 minutes
Cooking time: 15 minutes
Serves 2

INGREDIENTS

- 1 tbsp coconut oil
- 1 garlic clove, crushed
- 1 celery stalk, chopped
- 2 spring onions, chopped
- 600 ml vegetable stock
- zest of 1 lemon
- 200 g broccoli florets
- 1 tbsp fresh parsley, chopped
- 100 g spinach leaves
- 2 tbsp lemon juice
- 2 tbsp nutritional yeast flakes
- ½ avocado
- sea salt and black pepper

For the hazelnut sprinkle:
- 30 g hazelnuts, toasted and chopped
- 2 tbsp fresh parsley, chopped
- 2 tsp hazelnut or walnut oil

PER SERVING	
Calories	344 kcal
Protein	16.7 g
Total Fat	26.2 g
Saturates	6.3 g
Carbohydrates	10.2 g
Sugar	3.5 g

Heat the coconut oil in a medium-sized pan and sauté the garlic, celery and spring onions for 2–3 minutes.

Add the vegetable stock, broccoli and parsley, bring to the boil and simmer for 10 minutes. Stir in the spinach, lemon juice lemon zest, and nutritional yeast flakes and let the spinach wilt. Transfer the contents of the pan to a blender.

Add the avocado, season to taste and blend until smooth. Spoon into bowls.

To make the hazelnut sprinkle, mix together the hazelnuts, parsley and oil. Scatter the mixture over the soup to serve.

Frittata Traybake

This delicious frittata is a great breakfast, lunch or speedy dinner option.
You can use any leftover vegetables you like in this dish. It can also
be cooked in advance and served cold. Eggs are a nutritious option as
they are rich in choline, a phospholipid important for egg health and
foetal development. They also provide plenty of protein to support egg
and sperm development as well as to help stabilise blood sugar levels
throughout the day.

Preparation time: 15 minutes
Cooking time: 33 minutes
Serves 2

INGREDIENTS

- 5 eggs
- 60 ml whole milk or coconut cream
- 1 tbsp coconut oil
- ½ small red onion, diced
- 1 garlic clove, crushed
- 1 courgette, grated
- 100 g cooked vegetables (for example, sweet potato or carrot), cut into cubes
- 1 tbsp fresh parsley, chopped
- 2 tbsp Parmesan, grated
- sea salt and black pepper

PER SERVING	
Calories	376 kcal
Protein	24 g
Total Fat	27.6 g
Saturates	14.1 g
Carbohydrates	7.7 g
Sugar	7.1 g

Preheat the oven to 180°C (gas mark 4). Line a small deep baking dish or tin with baking parchment, making sure the baking parchment lines the sides as well as the base.

Beat the eggs in a bowl, whisk in the milk and season well.

Heat the coconut oil in a frying pan and sauté the onion and garlic until soft, about 2–3 minutes. Add the courgette, cooked vegetables and parsley and mix well.

Scatter the vegetables in the base of the baking tin. Pour over the egg mixture and scatter over the cheese.

Place in the oven and cook for 30 minutes until golden and the egg is cooked through.

Cool for a couple of minutes, then lift out of the tin and cut into portions to serve.

Chilli Sweet Potato Chips with Avocado Ranch Dip

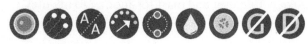

These lightly spiced chips are perfect for dunking into the deliciously creamy ranch dip. They are ideal as a snack or as a side dish to a main meal. You can use kefir or coconut kefir in dips and dressings as an easy way to cram in more beneficial bacteria, but if this is not available use yoghurt or coconut cream instead. Sweet potatoes are a great source of soluble fibre to support healthy blood sugar levels and digestive health.

Preparation time: 15 minutes
Cooking time: 25 minutes
Serves 2

INGREDIENTS

- 2 tbsp coconut oil, melted, plus extra for greasing
- 400 g sweet potato, cut into 1-cm thick strips
- pinch of red chilli flakes
- sea salt and black pepper

For the avocado ranch dip:

- ½ ripe avocado, chopped
- 1 tbsp omega blend, olive or walnut oil
- 1 tbsp kefir or coconut kefir, or coconut cream
- 2 tsp apple cider vinegar
- 1 tsp fresh parsley, chopped
- 1 tsp chopped fresh dill
- ½ tsp Dijon mustard
- ½ tsp garlic salt

PER SERVING	
Calories	350 kcal
Protein	3.2 g
Total Fat	19.4 g
Saturates	9.8 g
Carbohydrates	40.5 g
Sugar	11.4 g

Preheat the oven to 200°C (gas mark 6). Lightly grease a large baking tray with a little coconut oil.

Combine the oil, sweet potato strips and chilli flakes in a large bowl. Season with salt and pepper and toss to coat.

Spread the sweet potato chips on the prepared tray in a single layer. Roast for 10–15 minutes until golden. Turn over and roast for another 10 minutes or until soft and golden.

To make the dip, place all the ingredients in a blender and process until smooth. Season to taste. Place in a bowl and serve alongside the chips.

Raspberry Mousse Pots

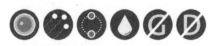

Deliciously simple and packed with protein, these are ideal as a healthy snack, dessert or breakfast option. The addition of acai powder provides plenty of protective antioxidants, while the coconut oil is a great source of healthy fats and lauric acid to support immune function. You can use bags of frozen fruit for ease or for when raspberries are out of season.

Preparation time: 15 minutes
Cooking time: 2 minutes
Serves 4

INGREDIENTS

For the crumble topping:

- 1 tsp coconut oil
- 30 g large porridge or gluten-free oats
- pinch of cinnamon
- 1 tsp maple syrup or honey

For the mousse:

- 50 g vanilla protein powder
- 1 tsp inositol powder
- ½ tsp acai or goji berry powder
- 225 g fresh or frozen raspberries
- 100 g coconut oil, melted
- 100 g macadamia nuts
- 1 tsp vanilla extract
- juice of 1 orange
- 30 g xylitol or honey
- ½ tsp probiotic powder (optional)

PER SERVING	
Calories	554 kcal
Protein	13.3 g
Total Fat	47.3 g
Saturates	25.3 g
Carbohydrates	21.5 g
Sugar	8.3 g

To make the topping, melt the coconut oil in a frying pan then toss in the oats. Stir over a medium heat and add the cinnamon and maple syrup. Cook for a couple of minutes until golden. Take off the heat.

For the mousse, place all the ingredients in a high speed blender and process until smooth and creamy.

Spoon the mousse into shot glasses or little bowls and top with the crumble mixture.

CHAPTER NINETEEN

Embryo Transfer and Implantation

In the days before transfer you will have had ongoing conversations with your clinic about how your embryos are developing. The day that transfer occurs is a big day for every couple undergoing IVF treatment. This can vary between 2 and 5 days depending on how many embryos have fertilised and the quality of these embryos. The higher the number of embryos available, the greater the chances of getting to day 5 blastocyst transfer. Having got this far is an achievement in itself, but it can also be a time of anxiety. (Note that if your embryos are transferred sooner than five days, you still have every chance of becoming pregnant.)

THE TRANSFER

For the majority of women embryo transfer is straightforward – feeling rather like a cervical smear (see page 26). The aim with most transfers is to put one good embryo back into the womb and to freeze any good remaining embryos. Older women may have more than one embryo transferred.

> If you've had any previous surgical procedures, your transfer may be slightly more complicated, and in this case your clinic may suggest that you have a 'mock transfer' before your IVF cycle begins to establish the best way to proceed.

There is much debate about whether or not women should rest after transfer. I believe that this is a tiring, stressful and emotional time for every couple and that a period of rest, with lots of sleep and lots of relaxation, is a good thing. However, if you want to (or have to) go back to work straightaway, there are no reasons that we know of why this shouldn't be okay.

USING YOUR DIET

This is a time for nourishing foods that will encourage good blood flow (the Chinese are great believers in foods that can nourish the blood) and improve your energy levels. Iron-rich foods, such as leafy greens, are a good start, as well as foods that are anti-inflammatory and those that will help to modulate your immune system.

IMPLANTATION

Whatever type of IVF you undergo, once the embryo has been transferred into your womb implantation is something the embryo and body have to do for themselves, when the embryo attaches to the womb lining (the endometrium) and starts to embed. Chemical messengers send signals between the embryo and the endometrium to allow implantation to happen.

The complex interplay of hormones and chemical messengers create a 'window of implantation' – the distinct period during which the uterus is receptive to receiving the embryo (or blastocyst) and allowing it to implant. A healthy implantation lays down the foundations for a healthy pregnancy – it can determine how the pregnancy progresses and have an influence over complications, such as pre-eclampsia and poor foetal growth, that may occur during pregnancy. Nourishing your body to assist implantation can help to protect you against such conditions and can lower your risk of premature birth.

THE IMPLANTATION PROCESS

In order to prepare for implantation, your body undergoes myriad changes. In response to the arrival of the embryo in the womb, the body produces raised levels of sugars (glycogens), fats (lipids) and proteins to fuel, support and build during the implantation process.

Amazingly, as it floats in your womb, the embryo 'talks' to the cells of your womb lining, triggering the release of certain hormones to enable the body to accept the foreign cells. There is a small window of only a few days when your uterine lining is prepared to accept the embryo and allow it to embed, so this communication – and hormonal efficiency – is key.

An incredibly complex, simultaneous production of proteins and sugars enables the embryo to shed its lining and to embed in the womb. It develops a protective layer of protein cells that permit the transfer of nutrients and water from the mother, but prevent the passage of her blood cells (which would trigger an immune response). Once the embryo has settled into position, its own cells and the cells of the endometrium begin to communicate directly, further influencing hormone levels (including raised progesterone) that allow the pregnancy to continue.

This is a very crude summary of what is an intricate, highly developed system that marks the beginning of pregnancy. You won't 'feel' pregnant at any time during this process and many women going though IVF take this as a bad sign. However, it's perfectly normal to feel 'normal' – it's the same for any woman becoming pregnant by any means. Try to remember that implantation is a time when your body is working away, silently but incredibly hard, to do its best to make the IVF cycle a success for you.

IMPROVING IMPLANTATION SUCCESS

Every year advances in medical science enable us to improve success rates in IVF. Here, Rob Smith, senior embryologist at CARE Fertility London, explains some advances that specifically relate to implantation, which could make your chances of having a baby even better.

There are two ways in which we have been able to improve the rates of IVF success through scientific advances. First, through improved embryo selection to ensure that only the best-quality embryos are chosen for implantation, and second through technologies that allow us to improve the likelihood that the lining of the uterus will receive the embryo successfully. For some women, even when good-quality embryos are introduced into the uterus, pregnancy doesn't occur. In fact, estimates are that implantation issues could account for up to two-thirds of failed IVF cycles.

During the normal course of the menstrual cycle, progesterone, released after the egg has begun its journey down the fallopian tube, signals to the endometrium – the womb lining – to thicken up ready to receive the fertilised egg. Only when the endometrium is at optimum thickness can the implantation occur. Although we can generalise about the few days in the cycle at which the endometrium will be at optimum thickness (in conventional IVF, this is set at being between days 5 and 7 in the cycle), every woman's cycle is slightly different, which means that general timings don't always produce the most desirable outcomes.

Technological advances, however, have allowed us to identify several ways in which we can improve implantation success rates for women who have had repeated failed IVF attempts, despite good-quality embryos being introduced to the uterus.

Genetic screening

In natural conception the body's own processes filter out embryos that might not make for a successful pregnancy or a healthy baby – these are embryos that show some genetic anomalies or chromosomal (genetic) defects. Of course, the process is not certain and pregnancy can occur even when an embryo has a chromosomal anomaly. In IVF we want to do everything we can to minimise the risks that a baby will miscarry as a result of a chromosomal anomaly and that means implanting the embryos that are least likely to have a chromosomal defect.

There are two types of genetic screening: pre-implantation genetic screening (PGS) and pre-implantation genetic diagnosis (PGD). In both cases, once the fertilised eggs have developed into embryos and are dividing and developing within the incubator, an embryologist removes some genetic material from each developing embryo and checks it for chromosomal anomalies. We are all made of 46 chromosomes, split up into 23 pairs – one chromosome from each pair comes from the egg and the other comes from the sperm.

Sometimes an extra chromosome appears on a pairing (for example, Down's syndrome is a condition caused by a grouping of three chromosomes, known as trisomy, on what should be pair 21). This causes a congenital abnormality or condition that may hamper the embryo's chances of implanting or may result in a life-limiting genetic condition for the baby.

Within an IVF cycle we are provided with the opportunity to check the number of chromosomes present in an embryo before putting it back into the womb (PGS). This will prevent specific, whole chromosome abnormalities developing in a subsequent pregnancy, such as Down's syndrome. Using a similar technology, we are also able to check for specific genetic mutations, such as the BRCA1 gene which causes breast cancer, and are therefore able to prevent it being passed through a family (PGD).

There are more than 250 PGD conditions currently listed on the HFEA's screening list. The question of what conditions can and can't appear on the screening list is both an ethical one and a matter of ongoing research – we don't always know the precise gene that causes a particular disease, disorder or condition. Presently the list allows for the screening for genes ranging from the BRCA1 and 2 genes that cause breast cancer and ovarian cancer respectively, to the various genes that cause haemophilia, early onset dementia and cystic fibrosis.

Time-lapse imaging

There's no getting away from the fact that genetic screening for embryos is risky – it requires an embryologist to remove cells at a very delicate stage of embryo development. Even simple observation of developing embryos requires them to be removed from the incubator once a day and looked at under a microscope. Time-lapse imaging, on the other hand, precisely measures the cell division using video techniques. A computer program analyses the video information according to certain cell-division parameters that embryologists know are relevant to embryo viability. It is completely without risk to the embryos, as the test doesn't require anyone to touch or move them at all.

The analysis is thought to be around 85 per cent accurate at predicting which individual embryo in a set is most likely to survive and sustain implantation.

Embryoscope

The embryoscope is another time-lapse incubation device. This device differs because it allows for the embryologists to manually make developmental measurements (morphokinetics) of the embryos without the aid of an automated computer program. Using live birth data from embryos, which have developed within the embryoscope, each individual laboratory develops their own algorithm to select the embryo most likely to form a baby.

Intracytoplasmic morphologically selected sperm injection (IMSI)

Of course, embryos are made from both an egg and a sperm. In some cases, getting the best-quality embryos means selecting the best-quality sperm in the first place. Intracytoplasmic morphologically selected sperm injection (IMSI) is a technique that uses a fantastically powerful microscope (up to 15 times more powerful than a standard microscope) to select sperm that are 'morphologically' best suited for successful fertilisation. Sperm with the best morphology – shape and size – are believed to have healthier DNA.

What does the best-looking sperm look like? Well, according to the guidelines of the World Health Organization, the best-looking sperm are 4–5 microns long and 2.5–3.5 microns wide, with an oval-shaped head. Once identified, the sperm that come closest to the 'perfect' criteria are individually injected into the available eggs just as with ICSI (see page 28).

Endometrial Receptivity Array (ERA) test

The cells lining the uterine wall have to be ready and willing to envelop the embryo and allow it to burrow deep enough to become properly nourished, and therefore multiply in cell numbers, grow a placenta and develop into a baby. In order for this to happen, certain genes in your own body have to 'switch on'. The Endometrial Receptivity Array (ERA) test involves taking a small sample of cells from the endometrial lining during a non-IVF cycle and working out whether or not the relevant genes in those cells have switched on.

Embryologists can establish from the results whether or not the endometrial cells are pre-receptive (that is, not yet ready to receive an embryo), receptive (primed and ready) or post-receptive (the window for implantation has closed).

Using data about your own cycle and the information received from the cells taken during the ERA test, clinicians can work out precisely when your genes switch on and when your endometrium is best placed for the embryo to be introduced into your uterus during your IVF cycle.

Good foods for transfer and implantation

- Foods for circulation – berries, citrus fruits, nuts, watermelon, cantaloupe melon, garlic, ginger, turmeric, oily fish, celery, nattō, tempeh, acai and goji berries
- Foods to modulate inflammation – see page 105

- Fermented foods – kimchi, kefir, sauerkraut, yoghurt, nattō, tempeh, kombucha
- Bone broths, stews and soups
- Protein-rich foods – lean meat, poultry, fish, beans and pulses

USING YOUR DIET

In light of all the important communication that's happening between the cells of the embryo and your own body, every nutritional (and lifestyle) thing that you have been doing during the build-up to this stage, and all your weeks of preparation, count. As the embryo burrows in, its outer cells begin to form the placenta, which will provide nourishment to the baby throughout pregnancy. Over the coming weeks, even in the very first few days of implantation, the baby's organs will be forming. With all this building work going on, you need plenty of protein, as well as foods that improve blood flow to your womb (see below) and antioxidants to support your immune system and protect both you and the embryo from free radicals (see page 79).

Foods such as beetroot are well documented for improving circulation, but all fruit and vegetables that are high in antioxidant vitamins and minerals are a good start (see pages 67–73) for improving blood flow. Whole grains, healthy fats and sources of iron (leafy green vegetables, lean organic red meat and so on) are also good circulation boosters.

If you haven't already, eliminate completely all stimulants and refined sugars during the implantation window – remember that these can wreak havoc with your hormone balance.

Make sure you get plenty of sleep at this time – the hormones that regulate your sleep–wake cycle also affect the release of your fertility hormones. Aim for at least eight hours a night. See pages 40–41 for more information on how to improve your sleep quality.

RECIPES FOR EMBRYO TRANSFER

Speedy Smoked Mackerel Pâté

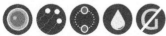

Mackerel is a fabulous source of omega-3 fats which are known to lower inflammation, improve sperm quality and the health of eggs and follicles. Aim to include two to three portions of oily fish in your diet each week. This is a simple store cupboard recipe and an easy way to cram more oily fish into your diet. Serve on rye bread with some sauerkraut or spread on oat cakes and accompanied by vegetable crudités. This pâté will keep in the fridge for three to four days.

Preparation time: 10 minutes
Serves 4

INGREDIENTS

- 2 hot smoked mackerel fillets
- 100 g cream cheese
- 100 g crème fraîche or Greek yoghurt
- 1 tsp freshly grated horseradish
- 2 tsp lemon juice
- 1 tsp fresh dill, finely chopped
- black pepper

PER SERVING	
Calories	382 kcal
Protein	10.8 g
Total Fat	37.3 g
Saturates	17.4 g
Carbohydrates	0.7 g
Sugar	0.6 g

Skin the mackerel fillets. Flake half of the fish into a food processor with the cream cheese, crème fraîche and horseradish and whizz until smooth.

Season with black pepper and lemon juice to taste, then fold through the dill and the remaining fish.

Place in a bowl, cover and chill in the fridge for 30 minutes to firm up slightly before serving.

Olive and Sun-dried Tomato Lamb Burgers with Barbecue Sauce

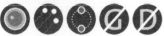

These tasty burgers are moist and flavoursome thanks to the addition of the olives and sun-dried tomatoes. Here they are accompanied by a deliciously tangy barbecue sauce and topped with lettuce and tomato. You can prepare the burgers ahead of time and keep them chilled until you are ready to cook. Where possible, choose grass-fed or organic lamb which tends to be richer in a valuable fatty acid known as conjugated linoleic acid (CLA). This fatty acid is known for its anti-inflammatory properties and may help with blood sugar balance. Lamb also contains plenty of sperm-friendly minerals, in particular zinc and selenium, as well as iron and B vitamins to keep the body energised. The barbecue sauce can be stored in the fridge for one to two weeks or frozen for up to three months.

Preparation time: 15 minutes
Cooking time: 12 minutes
Makes 4 burgers

INGREDIENTS

For the barbecue sauce:

- 75 g tomato purée
- 2 tbsp apple cider vinegar
- 1 tsp Dijon mustard
- 2 tbsp xylitol or honey
- pinch of smoked paprika
- pinch of cinnamon
- 1 garlic clove, crushed
- 4 tbsp tamari soya sauce
- sea salt and black pepper

For the burgers:

- 400 g lamb mince
- 4 sun-dried tomatoes in oil, drained and finely chopped
- 4 black olives, pitted and chopped
- 1 shallot, finely chopped
- 1 tsp ground cumin

PER BURGER	
Calories	538 kcal
Protein	41.9 g
Total Fat	33.3 g
Saturates	13.3 g
Carbohydrates	23.4 g
Sugar	7.8 g

- ½ garlic clove, crushed
  - a little coconut oil, for griddling

To serve:
- 4 wholemeal buns (optional)
- 4 lettuce leaves
- 1 beef tomato, sliced

To make the barbecue sauce, place the tomato purée, vinegar, mustard and xylitol in a small pan with the spice garlic and soya sauce. Bring to a simmer and cook gently for 10 minutes until the mixture has thickened. Season to taste and set aside.

To make the burgers, place the lamb mince in a bowl and add the tomatoes, olives, shallot, cumin and garlic and mix thoroughly. Season with salt and pepper. Divide the mixture into four and shape into patties.

Heat a griddle pan. Add the coconut oil and griddle the burgers for 5–6 minutes on each side or until cooked through.

To serve, split the buns in two, if using, and place a lettuce leaf on one half of each bun. Place a burger on each bed of lettuce and top with the tomato slices and a spoonful of the barbecue sauce. Finish with the other half of each bun.

Jerk Chicken Salad with Avocado and Mango Salsa

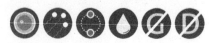

*The sweet salsa that accompanies this delicious salad is packed with
healthy monounsaturated fats and protein from the avocado and vitamin
C from the mango. Foods rich in vitamin C have been shown to improve
sperm quality and quantity and help protect sperm DNA from damage.
The spicy marinade is a perfect way to jazz up your salads, but is equally
delicious served with fish or duck.*

Preparation time: 15 minutes
Marinating time: 1–2 hours or overnight
Cooking time: 20 minutes
Serves 2

INGREDIENTS

For the marinade:

- ½ red onion, chopped
- 2 garlic cloves, crushed
- 1 red chilli, deseeded and chopped
- juice of ½ lime
- 1 tbsp tamari soya sauce
- 1 tbsp olive oil
- 1 tsp honey
- 1 tsp apple cider vinegar
- 1 tsp smoked paprika
- 1 tsp allspice
- ¼ tsp ground cinnamon
- sea salt and black pepper

PER SERVING	
Calories	283 kcal
Protein	39.4 g
Total Fat	8.7 g
Saturates	1.5 g
Carbohydrates	11.5 g
Sugar	8.4 g

For the salad:

- 2 chicken breasts, about 120 g each, boneless and skinless
- drizzle of oil
- bag of mixed rocket and spinach leaves
- 30 g black olives, pitted and halved
- ½ red pepper, diced

For the salsa:
- ½ mango, peeled and chopped
- 1 spring onion, chopped
- ½ red chilli, deseeded and chopped
- ½ avocado, diced
- 1 tbsp lime juice
- 1 tbsp fresh coriander leaves, chopped

To make the marinade, combine all the ingredients, except the salt and pepper, in a food processor and process to a smooth paste. Season to taste.

Place the chicken breasts in a shallow dish. Spoon over the marinade and coat the chicken thoroughly. Cover the dish tightly with cling film and marinate in the fridge for 1–2 hours or overnight, if possible.

When ready to cook, preheat the oven to 200°C (gas mark 6). Grease a roasting tin.

Place the chicken in the roasting tin, drizzle over the oil and roast for 20 minutes or until the chicken is cooked through. Cool for 5 minutes, then slice thinly.

Mix all the ingredients for the salsa together in a bowl.

To serve, place the salad leaves on a platter and top with the olives, red pepper and cooked chicken. Serve with the salsa.

Red Rice, Quinoa and Feta Salad with Pomegranate and Pistachios

Red rice derives its colour from anthocyanins, a group of potent antioxidants known for their protective properties. It is a good source of manganese, which aids the production of the compound superoxide dismutase (SOD), important for reducing oxidative damage and inflammation. Manganese is also useful for improving egg quality. Quinoa is high in protein and provides plenty of folic acid, iron, zinc and magnesium – all important nutrients for egg health. The perfect ingredients for a healthy rice salad!

Preparation time: 15 minutes
Cooking time: 25 minutes
Serves 2

INGREDIENTS

- 60 g red rice
- 60 g quinoa
- 1 tbsp coconut oil
- ½ red onion, sliced
- 1 small garlic clove, crushed
- 2 spring onions, thinly sliced
- 2 handfuls of rocket and baby spinach leaves
- 2 tbsp olive oil
- grated zest and juice of 1 orange
- 60 g feta cheese, crumbled
- 30 g toasted pistachios, chopped
- seeds of 1 pomegranate
- sea salt and black pepper

PER SERVING	
Calories	518 kcal
Protein	15.1 g
Total Fat	30.1 g
Saturates	10.6 g
Carbohydrates	44.2 g
Sugar	8.6 g

Place the red rice in salted water and bring to the boil. Simmer for 20 minutes until just tender.

Meanwhile place the quinoa in a separate pan and boil in salted water for 12–15 minutes until cooked. Drain and allow the grains to cool.

Heat the coconut oil in a frying pan and sauté the onion for 5 minutes until soft and lightly golden. Just before the end of cooking, add the garlic and cook briefly.

In a large bowl combine the rice, quinoa, onion and garlic. Stir in the spring onions, rocket and spinach. Whisk together the olive oil, orange zest and juice, and season. Toss through the salad. Gently fold in the cheese, pistachios and pomegranate seeds and serve.

RECIPES FOR IMPLANTATION

Beet Burst Juice

Energise your body during your IVF programme with this antioxidant-packed vibrant juice. Beetroots are a fantastic source of the antioxidant resveratrol, which is thought to help combat against age-related infertility. They also supply nitrates known to improve blood flow to the sexual organs making them useful for male fertility and for supporting a healthy uterus during embryo implantation.

Preparation time: 5 minutes
Serves 2

INGREDIENTS

- 1 large raw beetroot
- 1 carrot
- 1 celery stick
- 120 g fresh pineapple
- 1 apple
- 1 cucumber
- small piece of fresh ginger (optional)

PER SERVING	
Calories	80 kcal
Protein	2 g
Total Fat	0.5 g
Saturates	0.1 g
Carbohydrates	16.7 g
Sugar	16.6 g

Simply place all the ingredients in a juicer. Divide between two glasses and mix well before serving.

Health benefits

Beetroot provides plenty of folic acid in addition to nitrates. Your body converts nitrates into nitric oxide, a gas that widens your blood vessels improving blood flow and oxygen delivery to your organs. Use the core of the pineapple which is rich in bromelain, a digestive enzyme known for its anti-inflammatory properties.

Turkey San Choy Bau

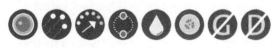

This Asian-inspired dish makes use of turkey mince to create a high-protein energising meal. Serve in lettuce cups and drizzle with a little sweet chilli sauce for a speedy nutritious lunch or dinner. Crammed with plenty of aromatic anti-inflammatory spices and herbs, this is ideal for a cleanse and for supporting the immune system. Shiitake mushrooms provide plenty of fertility-boosting nutrients, in particular selenium, B vitamins, zinc and manganese. They also contain polysaccharides known for their immune-modulating properties. Turkey provides plenty of easily absorbable iron, which helps to increase fertility, plus zinc and selenium important for male fertility.

Preparation time: 15 minutes
Cooking time: 8 minutes
Serves 2

INGREDIENTS

- 1 tbsp coconut oil
- 1 garlic clove, crushed
- 1 tsp grated fresh ginger
- 1 spring onion, sliced
- 300 g turkey mince
- 4 shiitake mushrooms, chopped
- 1 carrot, grated and peeled
- ½ courgette, grated
- 30 g bamboo shoots, cut into thin strips
- 1 tsp fish sauce
- 1 tbsp sweet chilli sauce
- 2 tsp tamari soya sauce
- ½ red chilli, deseeded and chopped
- a handful of beansprouts

To serve:
- 2 lettuce leaves
- 1 tbsp fresh coriander leaves, chopped
- 1 tbsp sesame seeds
- a little sweet chilli sauce, for drizzling (optional)

PER SERVING	
Calories	295 kcal
Protein	40.3 g
Total Fat	11.5 g
Saturates	5.4 g
Carbohydrates	7.4 g
Sugar	6.9 g

Heat the coconut oil in a large frying pan. Add the garlic, ginger and spring onion and sauté briefly for 1 minute. Add the mince, mushrooms, carrot, courgette and bamboo shoots and stir fry for 3–4 minutes until the turkey is cooked through. Add the remaining ingredients and stir fry for a further 2–3 minutes.

Divide the mince mixture between the lettuce leaves and scatter over the coriander and sesame seeds. Drizzle over a little sweet chilli sauce if desired and serve.

Chocolate Bean Brownies

Rich and fudgy, these delicious brownies are packed with protein thanks to the addition of cooked beans and protein powder. They are perfect as a healthy snack, on-the-go breakfast or as a pick-me -up when energy levels are flagging. The brownies can be stored in the fridge for one week or frozen for up to three months.

Preparation time: 15 minutes
Cooking time: 45 minutes
Makes 12 brownies

INGREDIENTS

- 60 g walnuts, toasted
- 60 g almonds, toasted
- 60 g pecans, toasted
- 350 g black beans, cooked and drained
- 60 g coconut oil, melted
- 50 g cocoa powder
- 1 apple, cored and chopped
- 60 g soft dates, pitted
- 50 g chocolate protein powder
- ½ tsp sea salt
- 1 tbsp vanilla extract

PER BROWNIE	
Calories	211 kcal
Protein	8.4 g
Total Fat	16.1 g
Saturates	5.8 g
Carbohydrates	10.6 g
Sugar	6 g

Preheat the oven to 180°C (gas mark 4). Line a 20 x 20 cm traybake tin with baking parchment.

Place the nuts in a food processor and process briefly until they are finely chopped. Add the remaining ingredients and process to form a thick soft batter.

Spoon the mixture into the traybake tin and smooth the surface.

Bake in the oven for 40–45 minutes or until cooked through. Allow to cool in the tin completely.

Cut into 12 bars to serve.

CHAPTER TWENTY

The Two-week Wait

This is the most difficult time for every couple going through IVF. For the woman in particular it can feel as though the body is playing tricks – some days you feel as though IVF has worked and you're pregnant; other days you can feel desperate that it hasn't and you're not. For most couples I see, the height of that stress –mixed with anxiety, anticipation and impatience – reaches its zenith during the two-week wait, the time between transfer and pregnancy test.

Women often describe this as an excruciating time – there is no active process to go through and nothing specific that anyone can do, it's just a question of sitting it out. For some it feels better to spend a couple of days recovering after implantation and then getting straight back to work – finding something to occupy the time. For others, the thought of being around people and having to behave normally is unfathomable. Women also often feel a huge sense of responsibility at this time – their partner has no input into this process and the onus is entirely on their own body to get everything right. For many women, who have been so intensely looked after at the clinic, this time can make them feel isolated and alone – there are no more appointments and there is no news that anyone at the clinic can tell them.

Or, at least, that's how they feel. Of course, in reality there are no right and wrong ways to behave or things to do at this stage. All you can do is take steps to ease your way through the stress and to support each other fully. Take a look at the stress-reduction techniques on pages 45–8 and try to fit in at least 20 minutes of dedicated relaxation every day. That might be formal relaxation techniques, such as time spent in visualisation or meditation, or it might be something else that you find relaxing – a gentle walk in the park, time sitting with your favourite book or listening to your favourite composer. Remember to call upon your support network at this time, for distraction if not advice – your friends and family will be happy to help you. And don't forget each other. Keep talking, treat yourselves to a cinema or theatre trip, have a meal out or visit a place that you both love.

Spotting

It's perfectly normal to experience some 'spotting' during the two-week wait, especially if more than one embryo has been transferred. Tell your clinic about it if it occurs, but remember that it doesn't mean you aren't pregnant. Don't stop taking your medication.

USING YOUR DIET

Alongside the nutrients suggested at the time of transfer (see page 211), if you are feeling a bit anxious and stressed, look at foods that are good for relieving stress (see pages 49–50), as well as supporting your nutrient intake through the way that you eat (see box below).

Most importantly of all, avoid junk foods, refined carbohydrates, refined sugar and saturated fats, and all stimulants (caffeine, for example). High-sugar snacks might give you an energy burst that makes you feel as though you're coping, but they will be quickly followed by a slump that will only add to any despair. Staying positive and staying calm means keeping your blood sugar levels stable – you can find out how on pages 152–3.

If I had to pick one stress-busting nutrient group to boost above all others, it would be the B vitamins. Stress eats up B vitamins, because your body uses them to try to regulate the metabolism and put things back into balance. B vitamins are also essential for the health of your nervous system, itself fundamental to your stress response. Whole grains are the best food sources of these nutrients, but you can also find them in seaweed and raw vegetables. Protein is also a good source so I advise that it's important to keep up protein intake at this time. Furthermore, stress depletes the body of antioxidants, including vitamins A and C and magnesium – boosting your intake of colourful fruit and vegetables will help get things back on track. Finally, make sure you get lots of good-quality iron in your diet (from nuts and seeds, as well as organic meat) – this will help your body transport nutrients around your system effectively, combatting the effects of stress on your body's systems.

Eight ways to support your stress-busting diet

Here are my top tips for supporting your stress-busting diet through the way that you eat:

1) Get at least eight hours of good-quality sleep a night (see page 40).
2) Include 30 minutes of exercise every day – you don't have to go to the gym but walking, swimming, etc. can all be helpful.
3) Eat your meals sitting at a table, concentrating on your food or on the conversation with the people you're with at the table, not on a screen – be it a phone, your tablet or the television – or even reading a book or newspaper. Make mealtimes about your meal. You can even use chewing as a focus for meditation (properly chewing also begins the process of breaking down your food, easing the pressure on your gut).
4) Get some fresh air every day, even if it's raining.
5) Eat at least two to three hours before you go to bed, and save your heaviest meal for lunchtime if possible (and make your dinner a light one).
6) Load your carbs earlier in the day (breakfast and lunch) and make your evening meal a protein-rich one.
7) Stay off Dr Internet! Use your human support networks and don't trawl the Internet looking for sites that list signs of being pregnant.
8) Avoid acupuncture at this time – just give yourself time to relax without treatment of any kind.

RECIPES FOR STRESS REDUCTION

Chaga Almond Cacao Shake

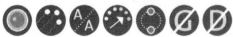

Chaga mushroom is known for its longevity-boosting and immune-modulating properties. Available as a tea, tincture or powder it is delicious when combined with chocolate in a drink. This creamy shake is packed with protein and healthy fats to help balance blood sugar. The maca powder helps nourish the adrenal glands too, making it an ideal drink to reduce the impact of stress on the body.

Preparation time: 5 minutes
Serves 2

INGREDIENTS

- 400 ml almond milk
- 150 g frozen pitted cherries
- ½ banana, chopped
- 2 handfuls of romaine lettuce, spring greens or kale
- 1 tsp chaga powder
- 1 tbsp lucuma powder
- 1 tbsp raw cacao powder
- 1 tbsp chia seeds
- 1 tsp vanilla extract
- 1 tsp maca powder
- 1 tbsp coconut oil
- 2 tsp almond nut butter
- pinch of ground cinnamon

PER SERVING	
Calories	274 kcal
Protein	5.6 g
Total Fat	13.3 g
Saturates	5.3 g
Carbohydrates	33.5 g
Sugar	12.8 g

Simply place all the ingredients in a blender and process until smooth and creamy.

Health benefits

Lucuma powder is a natural sweetener rich in fibre to support digestive health. Almond nut butter provides plenty of healthy fats, protein and vitamin E, known for its antioxidant properties and supporting egg and sperm health.

Seared Duck Breast with Orange and Star Anise

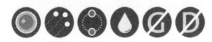

A delicious lightly spiced dish, moist and full of flavour, this would be perfect served with a tray of roasted seasonal vegetables or a simple mixed salad. Duck is an excellent source of protein and is rich in iron and selenium. Selenium helps to improve the body's immunity because of its antioxidant role. Along with other antioxidants, such as vitamins C and E, selenium helps to protect cells from free radical damage. It also provides plenty of the B vitamin niacin which helps to stabilise blood sugar and support energy production.

Preparation time: 15 minutes
Marinating time: 1–2 hours or overnight
Cooking time: 24 minutes
Serves 2

INGREDIENTS
- 2 duck breasts, skin on, about 120 g each
- pinch of dried chilli flakes
- 1 tsp ground cumin
- 200 ml orange juice
- 1 tbsp tamari soya sauce
- 1 tbsp balsamic vinegar
- 4 star anise
- 1 orange
- sea salt and black pepper

PER SERVING	
Calories	234 kcal
Protein	26.3 g
Total Fat	8.6 g
Saturates	2.5 g
Carbohydrates	13.8 g
Sugar	13.8 g

Score the duck skin 2–3 times without cutting through to the flesh. Rub over the chilli flakes and cumin and season well. Place the duck in a shallow dish. Pour over the orange juice, soya sauce and vinegar and add the star anise. Cover the dish tightly with cling film and marinate in the fridge for 1–2 hours or overnight, if possible.

When ready to cook, peel the orange and cut it into thin slices.

Heat a frying pan over a medium heat. Remove the duck breasts from the marinade and place them in the pan, skin-side down. Cook for 3–4 minutes, until the skin is golden brown and crisp. Turn and cook the other side for 3–4 minutes, then remove from the pan and set aside. Discard any excess fat from the pan.

Add the marinade to the pan and bring to the boil. Simmer for 5–6 minutes, until reduced by about half. Return the duck breasts to the pan with the orange slices. Cover the pan and simmer for a further 7–10 minutes until the duck is cooked through.

Remove the duck breasts from the sauce, place on a cutting board and leave to rest for 3–4 minutes. Slice and serve with the sauce poured over.

Caramel Chocolate Superbites

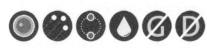

This is a healthy sweet treat packed with superfoods to nourish the body and help the body cope with stress. Maca and ashwagandha are well-known herbal adaptogens known to support the body during times of stress. The addition of protein powder ensures these bites will help support blood sugar balance as well as provide essential nutrients for egg and sperm development. These keep well in the fridge or can be frozen for up to three months.

Preparation time: 15 minutes
Freezing time: 30 minutes
Chilling time: 30 minutes
Makes 16 bites

INGREDIENTS

- 200 g almond, cashew or Brazil nut butter
- 2 tbsp honey
- 2 tbsp coconut flour
- 50 g vanilla protein powder
- 1 tsp cinnamon
- 1 tbsp vanilla extract
- 1 tsp inositol powder
- pinch of sea salt
- 1 tbsp lucuma powder
- 1 tsp maca powder
- 1 tsp ashwagandha powder
- 2–4 tbsp almond milk, water or whole milk

For the coating:
- 150 g sugar free dark chocolate chips
- 1 tsp coconut oil

PER SERVING (ONE BITE)	
Calories	156 kcal
Protein	5.5 g
Total Fat	9.5 g
Saturates	3.2 g
Carbohydrates	13.1 g
Sugar	7.5 g

Line a baking tray with baking parchment.

Place the nut butter and honey in a food processor and blend briefly to combine. Add the remaining ingredients and process until smooth.

With damp hands take walnut-size pieces of the mixture and roll into balls. Place on the baking tray and freeze for 30 minutes to harden.

To coat, melt the chocolate chips with the coconut oil in a pan. Dip the balls in the chocolate and place back on the lined baking tray. Chill for 30 minutes until firm.

Fig, Pear and Pistachio Muffins

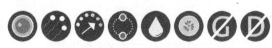

Figs have long been renowned for their ability to improve fertility and for boosting libido. Figs are rich in iron, which is important for healthy eggs and ovulation. Pistachio nuts are rich in healthy monounsaturated fats, L-arginine (important for sperm health), B vitamins and antioxidants including vitamin E – essential for protecting eggs and sperm from free radical damage. The use of ground almonds provides plenty of protein while maca powder is useful for supporting adrenal health. These muffins will keep well in the fridge for three to four days or can be frozen for up to three months.

Preparation time: 15 minutes
Chilling time: 30 minutes
Makes 8 muffins

INGREDIENTS

- 250 g ground almonds
- 60 g tapioca flour
- 1 tsp maca powder
- 1 tbsp baking powder
- pinch of sea salt
- 60 g coconut oil or unsalted butter
- 60 g xylitol
- 1 pear, cored and grated
- 1 tsp vanilla extract
- 3 eggs, beaten
- 125 ml kefir or almond milk
- 100 g dried figs, chopped
- 75 g pistachio nuts, chopped

PER MUFFIN	
Calories	440 kcal
Protein	12 g
Total Fat	33.1 g
Saturates	9.5 g
Carbohydrates	26.7 g
Sugar	10.6 g

Preheat the oven to 180°C (gas mark 4). Grease and line eight muffin tin holes with paper cases.

Combine the ground almonds, tapioca flour, maca powder, baking powder and salt in a food processor.

Place the coconut oil or butter in a pan with the xylitol and melt. Stir to dissolve the xylitol.

Pour the oil and xylitol mixture into the food processor along with the grated pear, vanilla extract, eggs and milk. Blend to combine. Add the figs and most of the pistachio nuts and briefly pulse.

Divide the mixture between the paper cases and scatter over the remaining nuts.

Bake in the oven for 25–30 minutes until golden brown and or until a skewer inserted in the centre of a muffin comes out clean.

Allow to cool in the tin for 5 minutes before transferring to a wire rack.

CHAPTER TWENTY-ONE

When IVF is Successful

At the end of the two-week wait, usually about 16 days after egg collection, you'll be asked to take a pregnancy test. Some clinics will ask you to come in for a blood test, others will be happy for you to use a home testing kit.

A successful test at this stage is the first hurdle to a successful pregnancy. Many women we see in the clinic are so convinced they won't get good news (especially if this is a second or subsequent attempt) that the first emotion they feel is shock and disbelief. Soon this gives way to feelings of utter joy, which then themselves give way to panic. Many of the women I meet know so much about infertility and are so comfortable with the processes involved in not being able to have a baby, that the thought of dealing with the anxieties of being pregnant (in particular, the thought that, after all this, something might go wrong) become overwhelming. Most couples want to keep their news to themselves at first, too, which (while sensible) often adds to the mounting sense of pressure.

However, your clinic is there to guide you through these anxious early stages and there are lots of proactive things you can do to feel that you are busying yourself and actively supporting your early pregnancy. Your IVF team will also advise you on what medication you need to take and for how long.

COPING WITH ANXIETY

Look at all the advice for coping with anxiety during your procedure and put in place measures to help keep you as stress-free as possible. Anxiety can be very difficult to manage, so it is important to practice any techniques that will help you manage. Rest a lot and consider counselling, hypnotherapy, acupuncture and specific relaxation or meditation techniques. Following the important dietary principles below for early pregnancy, look back at your stress-relieving dietary principles and make sure you keep eating meals that are good at keeping your adrenaline and cortisol levels under control and manage your blood sugar. (See pages 152–3.)

Calculating your due date

In order to work out your due date following IVF treatment, find the date two weeks before your egg collection. Your due date will be 40 weeks from that date. For the purposes of using a due date calculator (there are many of them freely available online), treat the date two weeks before your egg collection as the first day of your last menstrual period – and allow the calculator to do the rest.

Early pregnancy is managed differently privately and on the NHS. The most important thing at this stage is to get the support you feel you need; if you have had a history of miscarriage or complications you may be referred to an early pregnancy unit.

SUPPORTING EARLY PREGNANCY THROUGH DIET

In principle the women I see who have prepared for IVF have followed nutrition advice to the letter. Therefore, they are sometimes shocked that during those early weeks they start to eat badly and crave carbs and sweets and often can't take their supplement. Do the best you can as it will take time to get used to being pregnant and understanding what your body needs. Often that is carbs for energy in the early days. Remember if you have been preparing your baby doesn't rely on what it has in any one day but on your reserves of nutrients.

By the time you have your pregnancy test, you are in the early stages of pregnancy. This brings with it its own nutritional needs – your body now needs to sustain the pregnancy and nourish a growing baby. There are also certain foods that it's best to avoid during pregnancy and especially during the first trimester when the developing baby is at its most vulnerable.

The first thing to say is that becoming pregnant is not now an excuse to eat for two! Studies show that the calorific needs of a pregnant woman are barely increased during pregnancy and that in fact it's better to think of boosting the nutrient content of the calories you eat, rather than eating more. (The rules are slightly different if you have a multiple pregnancy.)

For the first few weeks of pregnancy, you can give your baby all he or she needs by making sure you eat a diet that is rich in good-quality protein (lean meat and poultry, eggs and pulses, and soya products once or twice a week only), that contains moderate amounts of slow-releasing wholegrain carbohydrates ('brown' bread, pasta and rice, for example), that is rich in B vitamins (remember that folic acid is a B vitamin and is essential for the proper neural development of the baby; see box below) and small amounts of healthy fats. Eating a rainbow of fruit and vegetables will ensure a full range of vitamins and minerals make it into your diet to support all your body's systems during this busy time. However, if you find yourself craving more carb-heavy foods, you don't need to panic.

Although some sources advise increasing your intake of calcium, others say that it's a myth that the baby 'saps' calcium from the mother's bones and teeth. Nonetheless, making sure you have good amounts of calcium-rich foods in your diet (dairy products, as well as some vegetables such as spinach; see page 70) will do no harm to you or the developing baby and may help with the development of your baby's bones.

The best food sources of folic acid

Folic acid is actually vitamin B9. It is essential for the proper development of your baby's nervous system and studies have shown that a deficiency in this vitamin in early pregnancy can lead to neural tube defects in a baby – that is a birth defect occurring in the baby's brain or spinal cord and leading to conditions such as spina bifida. It's so easy to boost levels of this crucial pregnancy vitamin in your diet (and I also recommend supplementation). Here are some good food sources:
- leafy green vegetables, asparagus, broccoli, cauliflower, beetroot and Brussels sprouts
- wholegrain foods, including brown rice and pasta
- pomegranates, avocados, oranges and strawberries
- chickpeas, kidney beans and black-eyed peas

The great news is that if you've been following the IVF diet, you will have already boosted levels of folic acid in your system, which makes it very unlikely that by this stage in the process you will be deficient. Keep up the good work!

Finally, it's not just vitamin B9 that's important for your baby's health and development – various other B vitamins are good for cell and gene development in the embryo, and energy metabolism and hormone balance for you. See page 68 for good food sources.

You may begin to feel tired, even during these early few weeks. Use your diet to regulate your energy levels, following the guidelines that provide a steady supply of energy-giving nutrients, outlined on pages 152–3. Importantly, don't reach for unhealthy snacks when you feel tired! Think instead of a hunger or tiredness pang as an opportunity to nourish and support your pregnancy – have a protein bar, some raw sugar snap peas or a piece of fruit for a snack. And keep up your water intake. Staying hydrated (water, well-diluted juice or fruit teas are best – avoid caffeinated drinks) is an essential part of maintaining your energy levels.

Early pregnancy supplements

You can buy specially formulated pregnancy supplements that provide the right levels of all the vitamins and minerals you need to support the early stages of gestation. Try to find one that has good levels of folic acid, as well as omega-3 fatty acids (which might be listed as DHA) and vitamin D. I have formulated my own pregnancy supplement, which you can purchase directly from the website: www.zitawest.com.

FOODS TO AVOID

Most women now know that there are certain foods it's best to avoid during pregnancy. Advice changes all the time, but use the following as the basis of things to cut out of your diet and then talk to your clinic and midwife for the most up-to-date advice.

Foods to avoid throughout pregnancy because of risks they carry for the baby include:

* Uncooked unpasteurised soft or blue cheeses (which carry the risk of listeria infection that can cause brain damage in an unborn baby). Cooked unpasteurised soft and blue cheeses are fine, though, as are any cheeses (soft or hard) that have been pasteurised.
* Mercury-rich fish, including shark, tuna, marlin and swordfish, which can cause nervous system damage in an unborn baby.
* Cured meats, such as salami or prosciutto, and undercooked meat (including steak that you would normally eat pink), because these may carry the toxoplasmosis parasite (you don't have to worry about foods that have been pre-packed, such as pre-packed ham, or frozen and then thoroughly defrosted, as the packaging and freezing processes destroy the harmful parasite).

* Organ meats and foods made from organ meats, including pâté, as these are high in vitamin A, which may cause birth defects in babies if consumed in quantities that are too high (a normal diet that avoids organ meats will provide adequate amounts of vitamin A for its health benefits and not too much to harm your unborn baby).
* Raw or semi-cooked eggs. (British eggs with the 'won' symbol on carry a very low risk.)

It's also important to say that the risks to your baby if you do inadvertently eat one of these foods are very, very small. Let your doctor or midwife know if you're worried, but it's important not to panic.

Finally, you don't need to avoid peanuts or other nuts, unless you yourself have an allergy to them. Nuts contain lots of wonderful nutrients to support your pregnancy and there's no firm evidence to suggest that eating them while you're pregnant is likely to increase the odds of your baby developing an allergy.

The HFEA requires that all clinics in the UK hold statistics about the outcomes of treatments. For this reason, your clinic will ask you to inform them when you have your baby and give details about your pregnancy and the baby's birth, gender and health.

CHAPTER TWENTY-TWO

When IVF Fails

Many couples who have had failed attempts at other clinics come to see us. It is so hard when, for so many of them, everything had gone according to plan at every stage of the process and yet pregnancy didn't happen. Often a couple is looking for answers as to why and how. They want to know what their options are now and what the next steps are. While the science of IVF treatment is important, we can offer them an integrated approach that works alongside their clinical protocols and looks at all aspects of their situation. There are two key things needed for successful IVF: a good embryo and good implantation. Many lifestyle and diet factors can have an impact on the process, so there is a great deal couples can do to improve their chances next time round.

> If your pregnancy test is negative, don't stop taking your medications unless your clinic advises you to. Following a negative test, you may need to reduce your dosages slowly and carefully, according to medical advice. Consult your clinic about the approach that is best for your situation.

WHY IVF FAILS

YOUR AGE

As we've already discussed, age is the biggest influencing factor in terms of your chances of IVF success. If you're over the age of 40, the health of your eggs and your body in general is essential for successful conception. Remember that there is so much you can do to help make sure that your eggs are in as good condition as they can be.

YOUR EGG RESERVE

Anti-mullerian hormone (AMH) and antral follicle count (AFC) tests (see pages 12–13) are the key to knowing how many eggs you have in reserve. A low egg reserve doesn't make IVF impossible, but it will dictate the course of your treatment and its likelihood of success. It's important to maximise your chances by looking at the key nutrients for egg health.

FERTILITY-INFLUENCING CONDITIONS
Depending upon the severity, certain underlying medical conditions, such as PCOS and endometriosis, may hinder the success of IVF if they are not treated. Under- or overactive thyroid and being anaemic (having low iron levels), having low levels of vitamin D or an autoimmune or clotting disorder can all affect your odds of success. Your clinic should work with you to understand whether one of these could have been the problem in previous rounds of IVF.

CHROMOSOMAL ABNORMALITIES
Age is, again, the biggest cause of chromosomal abnormalities in a developing embryo, which can lead to failure of the embryo to implant. Embryo screening is a technique that can occur before transfer (see page 208) and can help to ensure that your embryologist chooses only those embryos without signs of chromosomal abnormality to put back into your womb.

BLOOD-CLOTTING DISORDERS
Women who have blood-clotting disorders are more prone to miscarriage. Once the disorder has been diagnosed (there are lots of tests to help this process), you can have extra medications during your fertility treatment to help thin your blood to prevent clotting.

Focus on homocysteine

One reason why women develop blood-clotting disorders is as a result of raised levels of the amino acid homocysteine in the body. In some cases, raised levels are due to the presence of a genetic mutation – particularly one called MTHFR. However, by increasing your intake of foods rich in folic acid and supplementing with a form of folic acid called methylfolate, together with B6 and B12, you can help to keep homocysteine levels optimal (see the products at www.zitawest.com). Good food sources of folic acid include lentils, black beans, spinach, asparagus, romaine and cos lettuce, avocado, broccoli, mango and oranges.

WHAT YOU CAN DO IF IVF FAILS

First, think about how you prepared for this cycle and what you could do differently if you were to do it again. Look at every aspect of your lifestyle, including your nutrition, for both you and your partner. We see a lot of women with many previously failed IVF and reproductive immunology is often a potential issue, so we do blood tests to understand more fully whether a particular client might be affected.

YOUR IMMUNITY

An immune imbalance is often the first assumption for a failed cycle and while, in fact, it is a relatively rare cause of failed IVF, it is a possibility for a small number of women. If you have an autoimmune condition (including gluten intolerance) or some other known imbalance in your immune system (see pages 173–5), focus on eating an anti-inflammatory diet rich in immune-modulating foods, as well as boosting your levels of vitamin D, the workhorse of the immune system (see page 69). Remember there are many lifestyle triggers that affect the immune system, too, including stress.

Understanding miscarriage

Miscarriage (which means losing a baby before you're 24 weeks pregnant) is very common for pregnancy, regardless of how you conceived. Some women, who experience recurrent miscarriage, think that IVF might provide a way forward. However, in this case it's not getting pregnant that is the problem, but being able to sustain a pregnancy. I believe that an anti-inflammatory diet supported by all the principles of good nutrition, especially a diet that is rich in free radical fighting antioxidants, is key in helping women who suffer repeated miscarriage to prepare their body to sustain a pregnancy to term.

ECTOPIC PREGNANCY

Ectopic pregnancy occurs when the fertilised egg implants somewhere other than the womb lining, most commonly in the fallopian tubes. IVF does carry a slightly increased risk of ectopic pregnancy occurring. In this case, the embryo inadvertently finds its way into the fallopian tube and starts to grow there. Ectopic pregnancy will always end in miscarriage and maybe the loss of a fallopian tube, but significantly it can be life-threatening for the mother and this is why it is essential that if you experience any bleeding after transfer, you let your clinic know straightaway. The risks are small, but they do exist.

BEGINNING YOUR NEXT CYCLE

Starting again isn't right for every couple. If your first cycle has been unsuccessful, using the information you've learned from that cycle and trying to improve your treatment in a following cycle may help to improve your chances of success. The lessons your clinical team learn can give insight into more specific tests you might need the next time round or more advanced techniques for stimulation, retrieval and implantation. In circumstances when those lessons offer hope, many couples decide to have another go.

For other couples, and for couples who have tried several times without success, circumstances (medical, emotional or financial) may mean that the time is now right for them to explore other options for parenthood – perhaps using donor sperm or eggs, surrogacy or adoption, for example. Or perhaps it's time to live a fulfilling life as a couple without children, as so many people do.

If you do want to start again there are certain things you can do to that may improve your chances of success the second time round, as well as learning from your previous cycle and adopting all the healthy lifestyle and dietary choices you'd made previously. The first is to wipe your physical slate clean, helping your liver to clear out the residual synthetic hormones and so on from your system. There are several ways you can do this but you should have a plan of action:

* Do the two-week cleanse on pages 148–51 so that you can start your new treatment cycle from scratch.
* Try acupuncture, asking your clinic to recommend a practitioner who understands the specific needs of couples undergoing IVF.
* Seek help through counselling or hypnotherapy to help reduce your stress levels.

Appendix

COMMONLY ASKED QUESTIONS

I have been running the Zita West Fertility Clinic for 20 years and still, after all that time and through all the couples I've met, there are questions that take me by surprise. What this shows me is that every couple's situation – not just in terms of their fertility health, but in terms of their emotional and psychological processing of their situation – is completely unique.

Nonetheless, there are also many questions that show me that couples have common concerns when it comes to their treatment. Over the following pages, I want to highlight some of these and direct you to the parts of the book where you'll find information that will help to answer them.

HOW LONG DOES AN IVF CYCLE TAKE?

A full cycle takes about 28 days – roughly the same as a menstrual cycle. It's hard to give a precise length of time as your cycle is unique to you and will vary depending upon your particular protocol.

See pages 188–93 for a full description of the IVF cycle and its phases.

WHAT ARE THE SUCCESS RATES FOR IVF?

Every clinic will have its own statistics for each type of IVF (see page 24) and you should ask to see those statistics before you begin, especially if you are paying for your treatment. You can also look at the success rates for individual clinics on the Human Fertilisation and Embryology Authority (HFEA) website.

See www.hfea.gov.uk.

WILL IVF TREATMENT USE UP ALL MY EGG RESERVES?

No. Every natural menstrual cycle involves several ovarian follicles developing, but usually only one will reach full maturity and release an egg. The others die away. In IVF treatment, your medication protocol will encourage more of the follicles to reach full maturity and fewer will die away. The net result of the numbers of follicles you use up in each type of cycle (natural or IVF) is the same.

See pages 12–13 for information about how we test for egg reserves and pages 25–6 for how we stimulate your ovaries to continue maturing eggs.

WILL THE HORMONE INJECTIONS HURT?

Clinics use injections into the tummy or a nasal spray. If your clinic uses injections, don't worry – most of the injections are superficial and shouldn't be any more painful than, say, any vaccination you might receive. Some might leave a little bruising at the injection site that will clear up in a few days. Some are also more painful than others such as progesterone injections.

See pages 24–7 for more about the IVF stages.

DO THE SYNTHETIC HORMONES HAVE ANY SIDE EFFECTS?

There are some side effects associated with some of the hormones you'll take, including mild to moderate PMS-like symptoms. The most significant possible side effect is a condition called ovarian hyperstimulation syndrome (OHSS), which can occur when fertility drugs cause too many eggs to mature within the ovarian follicles: this is more common in women with PCOS. Your clinic will give you a full list of all the possible side effects of the medications you'll be taking and the signs to look for if something isn't right, so that you can make a fully informed decision about your treatment options.

See page 27 for more information about OHSS.

CAN I EXERCISE BEFORE AND DURING MY IVF CYCLE?

Exercise is an important component of a healthy lifestyle. However, for women going through IVF we recommend you choose moderate, gentle forms of exercise so that you don't cause excess stress in your body. Think walking, gentle cycling, swimming and t'ai chi. If, before your treatment starts, you need to lose weight, your doctor can give you a carefully devised exercise plan that will help your efforts to lose weight safely. Don't suddenly begin vigorous exercising if you're not used to it.

See pages 190–91 for more advice on exercise during IVF.

CAN I HAVE A SPA TO RELAX BEFORE MY TREATMENT BEGINS OR DURING MY TREATMENT?

Spa days before your treatment begins are a brilliant way to feel that you're looking after yourself – and before treatment you can enjoy them to the full. However, once your treatment begins, although the emotional and relaxation benefits of being in a calming environment will be so good for you, you'll need to avoid certain aspects of a traditional spa day. This includes avoiding steams jacuzzis and saunas, certain types of massage (see below) and aromatherapy oils. Gentle swimming and time relaxing by the pool, though, are certainly to be enjoyed.

See pages 45–8 for other ways to relax during treatment.

CAN I HAVE A MASSAGE DURING MY TREATMENT?

Massage is a wonderful way to reduce stress and, in the Chinese system of medicine, to free up blockages in your energy and restore a sense of balance. However, always see a registered masseuse with experience of massaging women going through IVF treatment. Your clinic should be able to recommend someone.

See pages 45–8 for information about complementary therapies that we believe most help women going through IVF.

WHAT'S THE BEST WAY TO REDUCE STRESS DURING MY TREATMENT?

Meditation, visualisation, hypnotherapy, acupuncture and other complementary therapies and techniques are all good, safe ways to reduce stress while you're undergoing IVF treatment. If the treatment you choose requires a practitioner (that is, it is practised on you), make sure he or she understands the nuances of IVF treatment and can work with you appropriately. Your clinic should be able to give you a list of registered practitioners in your area. Your diet can help your stress levels, too – concentrate on eating mood-regulating foods and foods that balance out your blood sugars.

See pages 43–5 for detailed information about ways to reduce stress using your lifestyle and practices, and pages 49–52 for ways in which diet can help moderate your stress levels.

IS THERE ANYTHING WE CAN DO TO IMPROVE THE QUALITY OF OUR EGGS AND SPERM?

Yes, so much! Every step you take to reduce stress in your lives, improve the quality of the nutrients in your body and improve your hormone balance helps to enhance the quality of your eggs and sperm. In particular, you can slow down the ageing process in your eggs through careful nutritional choices.

See pages 78–83 for more information about how to improve the health of your eggs and sperm using your nutrition; and pages 79–80 to help reverse the effects of ageing.

WHAT SHOULD I TELL WORK ABOUT MY TREATMENT?

What you share with other people is a matter of personal choice. Some couples choose to keep the fact that they are going through fertility treatment entirely to themselves or tell only close friends and family. Others share their experience with a trusted colleague or a boss, in order to make it easier to attend appointments without having to answer awkward questions. If you have an HR department, someone there can be a good first port of call if you don't want to tell the people you work with directly. HR should treat information you give them strictly confidentially.

See pages 36–8 about how to maintain your relationships with the people around you while you are undergoing treatment.

SHOULD I GIVE UP ALCOHOL AND CAFFEINE?

Yes. That goes for nicotine (cigarettes and e-cigarettes) and other recreational drugs, too.

See pages 34–5 for a fuller discussion of why stimulants are bad for your fertility.

WILL I FEEL DEPRESSED DURING MY TREATMENT?

Psychological response to treatment is different for every individual and couple. Often the thought of embarking upon treatment is far more overwhelming than being in the process itself. Your clinic will give you strategies to help you cope with the stress and strain of IVF and offer you counselling to prepare you for the pressure of the treatment cycles themselves, the distress of a failed cycle and (perhaps surprisingly) the shock of a cycle that succeeds. I strongly recommend that all my clients take up opportunities for counselling, as talking, sharing and understanding are important pathways to relieving the potential sense of pressure or despair. If you do feel deeply low, however, call your fertility nurse straightaway to talk about what support is available to you. Never suffer alone and in silence.

See pages 36–8 for how to build a support network.

HOW EXPENSIVE IS IVF?

The cost of IVF varies from clinic to clinic (and some couples may be eligible for a free cycle on the NHS in the UK). Establish how much each round of IVF is going to cost you with your chosen clinic before you begin and work out between you how many cycles you're prepared to undertake before running into financial difficulty.

See pages 20–21 for more about the financial implications of IVF treatment.

WHAT IF I DON'T STIMULATE?

If you're worried about this find a clinic that will do an anti-mullerian hormone (AMH) test for you, as this will give you an indication of how you're likely to respond to treatment and help your clinicians to decide the levels of medication you need before you begin. As a result, no stimulation at all is very rare.

See pages 12–13 for more information about the AMH test.

WHAT IF NONE OF MY EGGS BECOME FERTILISED?

Although there is a possibility that this can happen, no fertilised eggs at all is very rare. If it does happen for you, though, you will need to cancel this cycle of IVF and begin again, if that's what you decide to do. Your clinicians will talk to you about what alternative IVF methods you can use next time round to increase the likelihood that fertilisation will occur.

See pages 24–9 for a summary of the different kinds of IVF, including ICSI in which individual sperm are injected into individual eggs, 'forcing' fertilisation.

HOW MUCH REST SHOULD I HAVE AFTER EMBRYO TRANSFER?

Whether or not you need to rest is a personal decision and depends upon your circumstances. I believe that on the day of transfer you should take it easy. However, after that it is entirely up to you whether or not you go back to your usual routine or take more time with your feet up. Some women find it makes it easier to tolerate the two-week wait before taking a pregnancy test if they are able to keep busy.

See pages 224–6 about what happens after embryo transfer.

CAN I FLY AFTER EMBRYO TRANSFER?

Although there are no obvious reasons why you shouldn't fly once the embryos have been transferred to your womb, we recommend that you don't take to the skies just yet. However, this is an individual descision.

See page 224 for more information about how to pass the time during the two-week wait.

WHAT HAPPENS IF MY FIRST PREGNANCY TEST IS POSITIVE?

You'll need to let your clinic know your news and you'll be asked to repeat the test a few days later, continuing to take your medications in the meantime. Assuming another positive pregnancy test, you'll then have an ultrasound scan to confirm the pregnancy.

See pages 235–9 for more information about what happens and how to look after yourself during early pregnancy.

WHAT HAPPENS IF MY PREGNANCY TEST IS NEGATIVE?

You may be asked to retest a few days later, but if the second test is negative sadly this round of IVF hasn't been a success. Your medical team will give you time to digest the news and then set about working out what might have gone wrong and why, and discussing with you where to take things from here.

See pages 240–41 for more information on what can go wrong.

About the Zita West Fertility Clinic

Zita West is a midwife, acupuncturist and fertility specialist who has been helping couples conceive for over 20 years. Fifteen years ago she opened the Zita West Fertility Clinic, now a leading provider of natural fertility and IVF treatment in London with Dr George Nudukwe as medical director.

The clinic has pioneered a holistic approach to IVF, combining the latest in IVF technologies with a range of complementary therapies to prepare couples, both mentally and physically, for conception and a healthy pregnancy. The clinic has built its reputation on successfully treating couples who have failed IVF at other clinics and believes that its holistic, whole body approach is responsible for its high success rates.

The Zita West brand is one of the UK's leading providers of vitamins and minerals for conception, pre-pregnancy, pregnancy and following birth. Their products also include meditation downloads to prepare the mind for pregnancy.

For more information go to www.zitawest.com or follow Zita on Facebook, Instagram and Twitter. Zita also has her own fertility show on YouTube and has affiliated acupuncturists in the UK and Ireland www.zitawest.com.

Index